America's War on Sex

Recent Titles in
Sex, Love, and Psychology
Judy Kuriansky, Series Editor

AMERICA'S WAR ON SEX

The Continuing Attack on Law, Lust, and Liberty

Second Edition

Marty Klein, PhD

Foreword by Nadine Strossen
Former President, ACLU

Sex, Love, and Psychology
Judy Kuriansky, Series Editor

 PRAEGER

AN IMPRINT OF ABC-CLIO, LLC
Santa Barbara, California • Denver, Colorado • Oxford, England

Library of Congress Cataloging-in-Publication Data

Klein, Marty.
    America's war on sex : the continuing attack on law, lust, and liberty / Marty Klein ; foreword by Nadine Strossen. — 2nd ed.
        p. cm. — (Sex, love, and psychology)
    Includes bibliographical references and index.
    ISBN 978–1–4408–0128–0 (cloth : alk. paper) — ISBN 978–1–4408–0129–7 (ebook)
1. Sex—United States—History. 2. Sexual ethics—United States—History. 3. Sex and law—United States—History. I. Title.
HQ18.U5K645 2012
306.7—dc23   2011051702

ISBN: 978–1–4408–0128–0
EISBN: 978–1–4408–0129–7

16 15 14   2 3 4 5

This book is also available on the World Wide Web as an eBook.
Visit www.abc-clio.com for details.

Praeger
An Imprint of ABC-CLIO, LLC

ABC-CLIO, LLC
130 Cremona Drive, P.O. Box 1911
Santa Barbara, California 93116-1911

This book is printed on acid-free paper ∞

Manufactured in the United States of America

CONTENTS

ACKNOWLEDGMENTS

I am a fortunate fellow. Standing at the nexus of several dynamic, creative professions, I have met many extraordinary people. I am privileged to present a work that is liberally seasoned with their ideas. It is a pleasure to publicly thank them.

My sincere thanks go to Debra Haffner, Bennett Hasselton, Bill Taverner, and Larry Walters for reading and commenting on various chapters—frequently on airplanes or while writing their own books and columns, often on tight deadlines. Each of these incredibly accomplished people took the time to challenge me to write better, and to lavish praise on me when I did. Larry also gave me a crash course in First Amendment law, for which I will always be grateful. And I'll never tell another lawyer joke again.

Many others contributed comments and answered my endless questions. I am touched to have received wise and timely help from Bob Corn-Revere, Clyde DeWitt, Milo and Nancy Fencl, Matt Foreman, Rebecca Fox, Judith Hanna, Phil Harvey, Marjorie Heins, Mitchell Katine, Mark Kernes, Doug Kirby, Raymond Lawrence, Judith Levine, Ricci Levy, Greg Lukianoff, Barry Lynn, Donell McDonell, Robert McGinley, Jeff Montgomery, James Morone, Candida Royalle, Bill Smith, Brant Wenegrat, and Jen Heitel Yakush, very busy people all. Without them this would have been a less compelling book.

Nadine Strossen has honored me by taking this book seriously. Her energy, commitment, courage, and clarity have inspired me from the minute I discovered her many years ago.

"Intellectual posse" may sound pretentious, but it captures the respect and affection I have for the world-class thinkers who supported me before and throughout this process: Larry Hedges, Peter Lehman, Janet Lever, Larry Magid, Jack Morin, and Pepper Schwartz.

I am pleased to thank Michael Carrera, who defines the word "mensch"; Sandra Cole, whose affection is like a purifying flame; and Jim Petersen, whose lessons about combining social science, artistic writing, show business, and a wicked sense of humor I still value and turn to.

While writing the first edition, I told Cynde Moya month after month that I would need her research skills "very soon." When I finally gave her an entire manuscript to format, and asked for it back within a week, she dropped everything else in her life and prepared a handsome, very useful stack of pages. Gina Lepore provided excellent research assistance on the second edition.

I proposed writing this book over a decade ago, but agents and publishers assured me there was no market for it. Over the years I burned to write it, but often became frustrated and considered giving up. My friends (and veteran sexologists) Michael Castleman and Vena Blanchard never let me forget how much I needed to complete this book, and urged me to persist. They were right. I am grateful to each of them.

Thanks to Judy Kuriansky for bringing me to the attention of Debbie Carvalko at Praeger, and thanks to Debbie for recognizing the value of my work. Debbie's continued participation in the second edition was a key factor in my decision to undertake it.

My wise and dear friend Veronica Randall read every sentence of every chapter (except this one) at least once, alternately massaging and wrestling with many of them. As a result this book is easier to read, and so you and I are both very much in her debt.

I greatly appreciate my agent, Will Lippincott. In addition to being smart, effective, and committed to my professional well-being, he's a charming, urbane guy. And really smart.

Finally, I thank my wife Randi—who, just by being herself, did everything a partner could possibly do to help me write this. I may be the one who writes about the human race, but she is the one who understands it. Like I said, I'm a fortunate fellow.

FOREWORD

Six years ago I wrote a Foreword to the first edition of this book. I said it was important, scholarly, and perceptive.

This second edition is a recognition of that importance and perceptiveness. Marty's ideas about the War On Sex have been both valuable and prescient; his many concepts such as "phony categories," "public-izing of private sexual expression," and the "Sexual Disaster Industry"—not to mention the War On Sex itself—describe important socio-political phenomena that directly affect all Americans' civil liberties.

I was delighted, though hardly surprised, when the American Association of Sexuality Educators, Counselors, and Therapists honored the first edition as their Book Of The Year. I trust that this second edition will inform, inspire, and empower still more readers to face the challenges of America's continuing War On Sex.

—*Nadine Strossen*
November 2011

I am honored to write a Foreword to this important book by my longtime colleague in the civil liberties movement, Dr. Marty Klein.

The reasons I consider this book so central to core civil liberties concerns can be graphically illustrated through my own family history. My beloved father was born a so-called "half-Jew" in Germany in 1922, and therefore suffered horrific human rights abuses under Hitler, including in the sexual realm.

Until the day he died, my father was eternally grateful to the young woman who had been his first love, when he was a young man living in Berlin as the Nazis were rising to power. The Nazis had classified her as an "Aryan," so she was risking her own safety when she defied Hitler's strict anti-miscegenation laws and continued her relationship with my father. Meaningful as her love and loyalty were to my father, they couldn't protect him from being deported to the Buchenwald concentration camp. Ultimately, though, my father was liberated from that death camp by the American troops who saved him—literally one day before he was slated to be sterilized.

In short, I have the most profound personal stake in preserving individual freedom in the sexual realm. I owe my very existence to my father's last-minute rescue from a regime that denied such freedom, as an essential element of its overall human rights abominations.

To be sure, it has been a while since we have faced such extreme discriminatory, coercive measures in this country as those that my father faced in Nazi Germany. Nonetheless, anti-miscegenation and forced sterilization measures did constitute official U.S. policy until shockingly recently—1967, in the case of miscegenation.[1] Moreover, had it not been for constant advocacy efforts by organizations such as the American Civil Liberties Union (ACLU), and by individuals such as Marty Klein, we might well still be subject to such repressive measures.

We must have the historic humility to recognize that it is always far easier, with twenty-twenty hindsight, to criticize past abuses—especially if they occurred elsewhere—than it is to recognize their current counterparts in our own backyards. Accordingly, Marty Klein's book shines a welcome spotlight on the many public policies today that continue to stifle full and equal freedom of choice for all mature individuals in the essential arena of sexuality.

I hope that the next generation will look back on our laws that bar marriage between individuals of the same gender with the same incredulity and shame with which we now look back on the laws from two generations ago, barring marriage between individuals of different races.

In short, in the words of the ACLU's principal founder, Roger Baldwin, "No fight for civil liberties ever stays won."[2] That in turn means, to quote a statement that has been attributed to Thomas Jefferson, which is also an ACLU motto: "Eternal vigilance is the price of liberty."[3]

Marty Klein's book vigorously rises to the challenge posed by both of these rallying cries. He explains in vivid detail the ongoing struggles to maintain freedom and equality concerning the whole spectrum of rights in the sexual realm: from the right to convey and receive medically accurate information about sexual matters; to the right to make our own choices about such fundamental, personal matters as contraception, abortion, and our sexual partners and intimacies. By documenting the mounting assaults on these essential rights, Marty is not only maintaining "eternal vigilance" himself, but also galvanizing all of you readers to do likewise.

In recent years, we have made some great strides forward in securing some rights regarding sexuality. For example, the Supreme Court has issued two pathbreaking decisions protecting the rights of lesbians and gay men,[4] and the Court also has consistently protected freedom for sexually oriented expression in various "new media," including the Internet and cable television.[5] I note these positive developments not at all to suggest that we should rest on our laurels, content with the progress we have made. To the contrary, I note the progress we have made, through education and advocacy, in the hope of encouraging all readers to raise their valued voices to help further these ongoing efforts. Marty's book is itself a valuable contribution to the ongoing struggles, and I share his hope and belief that it will in turn spur others to make their own contributions.

From my dual perspectives as a constitutional law professor and civil liberties advocate, the most important recent positive development was the Supreme Court's landmark 2003 ruling in *Lawrence v. Texas*.[6] In that case, the Court not only struck down the statute that was directly at issue—Texas's discriminatory ban on "sodomy" (oral or anal sex) only when it took place between same-gender couples. Additionally, of even more enduring consequence, the Court based its holding on broad-ranging libertarian and egalitarian rationales, which should sound the death-knell for other laws that restrict other personal conduct by consenting adults in the privacy of their homes.

Significantly, the *Lawrence* Court reversed its infamous 1986 decision in *Bowers v. Hardwick*, in which the ACLU had challenged Georgia's law that criminalized all "sodomy," or oral or anal sex, even between consenting adults in the privacy of their own homes.[7] In *Bowers*, the Court had held that government may criminalize private, consensual adult conduct, which inflicts no harm on anyone, merely because the majority of the community disapproves of the conduct. This reminds me of H.L. Mencken's famous definition of Puritanism: "the haunting fear that someone, somewhere, may be happy"![8] Seriously, it is hard to think of any purported justification for criminal laws that is more antithetical to individual liberty.

Let me quote John Stuart Mill's classic 1859 essay, "On Liberty":

> Over himself, over his own body and mind, the individual is sovereign. . . . [T]he only purpose for which government may rightfully exercise power . . . over anyone is to prevent harm to others. His own good, either physical or moral, is not a sufficient warrant.[9]

This famous statement well captures the bedrock civil libertarian premise that undergirds the ACLU's opposition to all laws that restrict the voluntary sexual choices of mature individuals. Indeed, this core concept of liberty is so fundamental that it also undergirds many other aspects of the ACLU's overall mission: to defend all fundamental freedoms for all people. One member of the ACLU's National Board put it very well, years ago, when we were reaffirming our opposition to criminalizing drug use by consenting adults. As he said, "When it comes to their own bodies, all adults have the right to imbibe, ingest, inhale, or insert whatever they want, wherever they want!"

The Supreme Court's opinion in *Lawrence v. Texas* contains language that celebrates a similarly broad concept of individual freedom of choice generally, and I find this especially exciting given that it was written by Justice Anthony Kennedy—a conservative, Republican, Catholic who was appointed by a conservative, Republican president, Ronald Reagan.

At the outset of his *Lawrence* opinion, Justice Kennedy ringingly recognized that constitutionally protected "liberty" encompasses not only the freedom to choose the particular kinds of sexual intimacy that were at issue in the *Lawrence* case—oral or anal sex with a same-sex partner—but also sexual intimacy in general. As he declared: "Liberty presumes an autonomy of self that includes freedom of thought, belief, expression, and certain intimate conduct."[10] It is noteworthy that Justice Kennedy ranks this constitutionally protected sexual freedom along with the time-honored First Amendment freedoms of "thought, belief, and expression," which long have been deemed so signally important that some Justices and other legal experts have called them "preferred rights."[11]

Not only does Justice Kennedy's opinion for the Court begin with an encomium to sexual freedom that would be worthy of Marty Klein himself, but Justice Kennedy concludes his opinion by eloquently endorsing the concept of a living, evolving Constitution in words that are worthy of the most liberal judicial activists. He proclaimed:

> Had those who drew and ratified the Due Process Clauses ... known the components of liberty in its manifold possibilities, they might have been more specific. [But] [t]hey did not presume to have this insight. They knew times can blind us to certain truths, and later generations can see that laws once thought necessary and proper in fact serve only to oppress. As the Constitution endures, persons in every generation can invoke its principles in their own search for greater freedom.[12]

One aspect of the *Lawrence* decision is of special significance in our ongoing struggle for rights respecting sexuality, which Marty Klein so compellingly documents. In overturning *Bowers*, the Court expressly held that laws criminalizing sexual conduct or expression cannot constitutionally be based only on majoritarian views about morality. This holding provoked the fiercest tirade in Justice Scalia's strident dissent. He rightly recognized that this holding should doom a whole host of statutes that now outlaw certain sexual choices, far beyond the discriminatory anti-sodomy statutes that were at issue in *Lawrence* itself. While these sweeping implications of *Lawrence* were the cause of Justice Scalia's consternation, for civil libertarians they are cause for celebration! As Justice Scalia wrote:

> State laws [that are only based on moral choices include laws] against . . . bigamy, same-sex marriage, adult incest, prostitution, masturbation . . . fornication, bestiality, and obscenity. . . . Every single one of these laws is called into question by today's decision. . . . This [decision] effectively decrees the end of all morals legislation.[13]

Make no mistake about it; it will take a long, hard struggle to realize fully the liberating, equalizing potential of the *Lawrence* decision, just as it has taken a long, hard—and still ongoing—struggle to realize fully the liberating, equalizing potential of the Constitution itself. But I always like to stress the positive. So although we are now facing increasingly strong assaults on our freedoms in the realm of sexuality—as *America's War On Sex* underscores— we must take heart from the fact that we also have increasingly strong tools to combat these assaults.

That said, it is always a struggle to persuade lower court judges and other government officials to actually enforce Supreme Court decisions upholding constitutional rights. Just as the Constitution itself is not self-executing, the same is true of Supreme Court decisions that enforce the Constitution. Often these are honored in the breach and require much litigation, including more Supreme Court rulings, to translate them into real rights for everyone, all over the country.

Just think of the long struggle, still not over, to fulfill the promise of the Supreme Court's landmark ruling against "separate but equal" public education in *Brown v. Board of Education*,[14] issued more than half a century ago.

Likewise, in the almost three years since the Court issued its landmark ruling in *Lawrence v. Texas*, we have had many disappointments, when lower court judges have read that decision as if it had no implications for any factual situation other than the one that was directly at issue in that very case.

And so, as Marty Klein's powerful book reminds us, despite civil libertarians' winning of such key battles as the one that resulted in the high court victory in *Lawrence*, the larger war goes on. At stake are all civil liberties connected with sexuality, in contexts ranging from A to Z—or, to cite two specific examples from both ends of the alphabet, from "abstinence" to "zoning." In citing abstinence, I am referring to the increasingly prevalent abstinence-only sex "education" programs in public schools, mandated by federal and state laws, which censor medically accurate information, thereby endangering the health and even lives of our nation's young people. In citing zoning, I am referring to laws that discriminatorily exile from our communities any businesses that engage in sexual expression, including bookstores that specialize in materials for the LGBT community.

Yes, my view has been shifting back and forth between two equally plausible perspectives: one that sees the glass as half-empty, by focusing on the ongoing War on Sex, and the other that sees the glass as half-full, by focusing on the defensive campaigns that have been successfully waged in that war, as well as the tools that these victories have provided to reinforce the continuing defense.

As an activist I am perforce an optimist, so I would like to close with the glass half-full perspective, quoting a key passage from a leading Supreme Court victory in this area. The passage comes from the Court's 1992 ruling that reaffirmed a woman's constitutional right to choose whether to carry her pregnancy to term, *Planned Parenthood v. Casey*,[15] in which the ACLU represented Planned Parenthood.

This excerpt explains why decisions not only about childbearing, but also about other aspects of our sexual and family lives, should remain in the private realm, for all mature individuals to resolve on our own, free from the heavy hand of government.

Significantly, this passage appears in the opinion that was jointly authored by three Republican Justices who were appointed by conservative, Republican presidents: Justices Sandra Day O'Connor and Anthony Kennedy, who were appointed by President Ronald Reagan, and Justice David Souter, appointed by the first President Bush. They declared:

> Our law affords constitutional protection to personal decisions relating to marriage, procreation, contraception, family relationships, childrearing, and education. . . . Our precedents "have respected the private realm of family life which the state cannot enter." These matters, involving the most intimate and personal choices a person may make in a lifetime, choices central to personal dignity and autonomy, are [also] central to [constitutionally protected] liberty . . . At the heart of liberty is the right to define one's own concept of existence, of meaning, of the universe, and of the mystery of human life.[16]

All of us who share the inspiring vision of Justices O'Connor, Kennedy, and Souter about "the heart of liberty" should be heartened by Marty Klein's book. It should encourage us to do whatever we can, both as engaged citizens and in whatever walk of life we pursue, to help transform this vision into a reality that is equally enjoyed by everyone.

Nadine Strossen[17]
President, American Civil Liberties Union
Professor of Law, New York Law School
New York, New York
April 13, 2006

INTRODUCTION TO SECOND EDITION: FROM BUSH TO OBAMA— LITTLE OR NO RELIEF FROM THE WAR ON SEX

BASELINE: BUSH

As documented in the first edition, the presidency of George W. Bush was a continual series of assaults and new restrictions on sexual rights. During this period America struggled through:

- The congressional pursuit of Internet censorship.
- The creation of the Department of Justice's Obscenity Prosecution Task Force.
- Massive funding of dangerous, inaccurate abstinence-only sex education, totaling over $1 billion.
- A dramatic reduction in reproductive rights.
- Multiple lawsuits, punitive actions, and regulations launched by the Federal Communication Commission (FCC) against "indecency" on TV and radio.
- Fierce maintenance of laws excluding homosexual men and women from military service, adoption, marriage, and other civil rights that the government routinely provides heterosexual Americans.
- Enhanced government cooperation with, and financial support of, "decency" groups such as Morality in Media, Enough Is Enough, Family Research Council, Concerned Women for America, and Focus on the Family.
- Increased state and municipal government interference with the rights of sexual privacy, assembly, and commerce. Successful targets

included sexually explicit magazines and videos, strip clubs, adult bookstores, revealing swimsuits, swing clubs, bathhouses, and even adult sex education centers.

ENTER OBAMA

The election of Barack Obama in 2008 was supposed to change many things, including government intrusion into private life. In the area of sexual rights, unfortunately, the positive effects have been extremely limited. More than halfway through Obama's first (and perhaps only) term, we can see several clear socio-political trends, including:

- Abdication of federal leadership in maintaining or developing sexual rights.
- Continued legislative ignorance (local, state, and congressional) about how the First Amendment and other protections of free expression relate to sexuality..
- Continued legitimacy of scare tactics, inaccurate beliefs, ideological agendas, and false assertions to justify virtually any legislative restriction on sexual rights.
- Continued expansion of government tools to undermine sexual rights, including zoning, eminent domain, police power, redevelopment, public health imperatives, exclusion zones, Sexually Oriented Business laws, bogus secondary effects doctrines, and medical regulations.
- Use of the Patriot Act and "national security" considerations to undermine sexual rights.

Lacking a clear vision or mandate from Washington, and with the president's bully pulpit disused and in tatters, individual states have aggressively led the way in increasing restrictions on sexual rights and sexual expression. Examples include restrictions on access to abortion, pointless expansion of sex offender registries with increasingly punitive conditions, restrictions on the availability of adult entertainment, protections for licensed medical personnel who reject their professional responsibilities, and heightened entrapment programs (often motivated by federal grants) to pursue adults in adult chatrooms engaged in fantasy age-play.

In addition, many sex-negative narratives or beliefs (all demonstrably false) have become more popular in American society during the Obama administration. These include:

- Sex trafficking is an enormous problem and is getting worse.
- Adult use of legal, adult pornography is a public health menace.

- The Internet is increasingly full of predators preying on young people.
- Sex research is a waste of time and money.
- Adults should be allowed to opt out of virtually any contact with sex-uality they find distasteful, whether in school (various sexual books, words, and ideas), at work ("conscience clauses" for pharmacists and others), in professional training (most medical students are no longer required to learn a full range of gynecological procedures), or in public (public art is increasingly sanitized of sexual content, including classic Greek sculpture)

Such discourses continue to complicate progressive efforts to base public policy on fact and science rather than on emotion and opinion. As the media, Religious Right, and conservative politicians continue to trivialize science as one perspective out of many—that is, just an opinion—it is increasingly diffi-cult to find legitimate venues with which to counter baseless anti-sex rhetoric with fact. The life-saving, virtually risk-free vaccine Gardasil is an example.

RELIGION

One of the most troubling aspects of the Obama presidency, and contem-porary state and local politics, is the continued exceptionalism regarding reli-gious belief in political life. Even more than under President Bush, religious sensitivities have a special seat at virtually all public policy tables, from repro-ductive rights to tax codes to employment policies.

Obama has actually expanded the destructive Office of Faith-Based Fund-ing begun by his predecessor. He started by naming Pentacostal pastor Joshua DuBois to lead the White House faith office (DuBois still holds this posi-tion). Obama then poured billions of dollars in federal money into social ser-vice programs that, because they are "faith-based," are exempt from the normal federal requirements of non-discrimination in hiring, firing, proselyt-izing, and so on.[1] When campaigning in 2008, Obama promised he wouldn't tolerate such discrimination, but he has and he continues to do so.[2]

Today's federal Department of Health and Human Services has reaffirmed that even health workers who are licensed to provide medical care are not required to perform their duties if their "conscience" instructs them not to. This is in clear contrast to anyone who declines to do their job if they believe Napoleon or Cleopatra instructs them not to. Favoring religious "instruc-tions" over non-religious "instructions" is a clear violation of America's invaluable separation of Church and state.

Virtually all instances of these religious fits of "conscience" involve sexuality—often reproductive services such as filling prescriptions for contraception, provid-ing D&Cs, performing abortions, and so on. The door is wide open for taxi drivers, janitors, office workers, and virtually any employee to claim a religious exemption from doing work that supports sexual expression with which a worker disagrees.

America's tax codes are quite clear in requiring that, in exchange for massive tax exemptions, religious institutions are barred from directly participating in election campaigns. Unfortunately, there are dramatic, ongoing violations of this regulation under the Obama administration. Thus, churches are now firmly part of the infrastructure that helps elect candidates who oppose reproductive choice and contraceptive access. Having been thus emboldened, the Alliance Defense Fund is actively campaigning to end this restriction on tax-supported Churches.[3] For more on this, see Chapter 13.

SUMMARY

So why have sexual rights become increasingly tenuous during this nominally Democratic presidency?

Part of the reason is the lack of a coherent vision of either sexual rights or sexual health coming from the president. One is tempted to excuse this by noting the profound systemic challenges this president faces—global economic collapse, enormous unemployment, a Republican Party focused solely on destroying his ability to govern.

However, the criminalization and sanction of ordinary sexual behavior causes great suffering for millions of Americans. To a parent who loses custody of her child because she's into sadomasochism (S/M), or a teen put on a life-long sex offender registry for texting nude photos of himself, the War on Sex is no abstraction that can be sacrificed to other issues. For people whose lives are damaged or ruined because of it, the War on Sex is real and current and profound.

Another reason the War on Sex has gotten worse is that the Religious Right has become stronger, smarter, richer, and more aggressive with regard to sexuality. Having almost completed its planned criminalization of abortion, it is now going after contraception and other medical interventions. They have successfully marginalized the wonder drug Gardasil, which could have protected an entire generation from human papillomavirus (HPV)—on the grounds that it "might" lead to "promiscuity." Indeed, it became an issue in the recent Republican presidential nomination process, as Michele Bachmann and others went after Rick Perry, who as Texas governor required the inoculation of schoolgirls several years ago.[4]

Finally, the Religious Right has created coalitions on zoning boards, city councils, and state legislatures that have reduced or even eliminated adult entertainment in large parts of the country. They have persuaded many major hotel chains to stop offering adult movies in guest rooms. Regional bigots like Phil Burress have been rewarded and are now national bigots.

A BRIGHT SPOT

In all, the outlook for sexual rights in America is dim, particularly with the leadership of the Republican Party jostling each other to prove that they are the most conservative, most religious, most anti-sexual, and least respectful of individual rights. This is a movement that demands small government—except when it comes to limiting Americans' sexual rights.

The only bright spot ahead in this regard is the dramatic advance in civil rights for America's lesbians and gay men. For more on that, see the Epilogue. For an update on everything else, turn the page.

Chapter One

YOU'RE THE TARGET:
WHY A WAR ON SEX?

The familiar expression *culture war* is part of the problem.

It suggests two sides of equal strength lined up in a series of battles, honoring more or less the same rules of engagement, wanting to conquer each other.

But what we commonly call the culture war is not like this at all. Those who fear and hate sexuality (erotophobes) are attacking those who appreciate or tolerate sexuality (erotophiles). And while erotophiles are *not* attempting to force erotophobes to live more sexually adventurous lives, erotophobes insist that both sides—*everyone*—live according to their erotophobic values. Erotophiles say, "If you don't want to go to a nude beach, don't go, but don't shut it down to prevent me from going." Erotophobes say, "I don't want to go to a nude beach, and I don't want you to have the option of going either. It should be closed."

While erotophobes acknowledge this recurring theme—that there's a huge range of opportunities for erotic stimulation, satisfaction, and imagination that they want to deny *everyone*, not just themselves—erotophobes also claim, paradoxically, that they are victims.

They say they are the ones who are tired of being attacked, their values and way of life undermined. Through so-called indecent entertainment, changing fashions, easy Internet access, a range of contraceptive technologies, and the occasional court decision, they say they are being force-fed sex. They can't, they say, turn on a TV, go to a mall, boot up a computer, or even go to work without being assaulted by sexual images. And that when they aren't being confronted literally, they are still forced to abide others' private sexual activity next door and all over America—behavior that is immoral, disgusting, and sinful.

This is, undoubtedly, true for them—*but irrelevant to the governance of America.* Nowhere in our founding documents is there any mention of regulating anything considered immoral, disgusting, or sinful. In fact, the United States was founded on the idea that people could choose what to do and with whom to associate based on their *personal* values and ideals—not those of a king, feudal lord, or religious hierarchy. Nor even, as James Madison declared, a tyrannical majority in their own town, state, or country.

When our fellow citizens say they want to eliminate entertainment, fashion, medical technology, bedroom activity, and businesses that are "immoral" or "sinful," they are calling for a dramatic shift in American law. Such major changes in the rules of American life would bring us far closer to modern Saudi Arabia, the former Soviet Union, Taliban-era Afghanistan, and Nazi Germany.

Historically, American society has tried to balance the needs of individual freedom and community responsibility. And so you can't yell "fire" in a crowded theater. Another fundamental American principle is that the law should address actual crime and actual victims, and it should be drafted in ways that limit unwanted or unanticipated consequences when solving a problem.

Today's War on Sex seeks to change this balance, and it has already succeeded in many ways. Historically, it was against the law for someone to *actually* kill your cow; now it's as if there's also a law against someone *thinking* about killing your cow, or doing something that makes you *worried* about someone killing your cow. And so attempting to criminalize abortion, for example, isn't enough for conservatives; now they are trying to prevent availability of emergency contraception, saying wider distribution would "encourage promiscuity." Liberals rush in with scientific data that clearly shows it won't, and one more battle is joined. As is common, the erotophobes have no data with which to counter—but they do have "concerns" and "feelings," *which are now considered seriously in public policy debates.*

We must ask directly: So what if a medication *does* encourage promiscuity? In a country devoted to individual choice, this shouldn't be a problem. And yet sexual jihadists have actually made this a consideration in American policy debates. The latest example is their successful attempt to block preteen girls from getting the HPV vaccine that would prevent cervical cancer. The Religious Right and "morality" groups don't claim the vaccine doesn't work, just that it will make teens less scared of sex (?) and thus promote "promiscuous" behavior.

Although our modern country requires drivers to wear seatbelts in case of accidents, has school athletes wear helmets in case they fall awkwardly, and establishes poison centers in case toddlers get into cleaning supplies, erotophobes *don't* want to reduce the consequences of unauthorized, unprotected, or unwise sex. They say that doing so encourages bad sexual choices. That's like saying seat belts encourage dangerous driving, and poison centers encourage sloppy parenting.

The politically powerful in America know that if you can get people looking at the wrong questions, it doesn't matter *what* answers they come up with. And so those who are trying to "clean up" America say they're fighting for a number of critical reasons: children, the family, marriage, morals, education, community safety. And now they argue that their actions promote "fiscal responsibility." But none of this is true. *It's really a war against sexuality:* sexual expression, sexual exploration, sexual arrangements, sexual privacy, sexual entertainment, sexual health, sexual safety, sexual imagination, sexual pleasure. Sexual *options.*

Most Americans care about their children, families, morals, and community safety. They are, understandably, easily drawn into a social conflict using terms like these, focused on the things that matter to them and about which they often feel powerless or confused. And so religious and other conservatives have Americans lined up behind them fighting a war that is not in their best interest. *The public is manipulated into fighting sexual expression, not sexual ignorance or poor sexual decision-making.* It then supports public policy that often defeats its own ostensible purpose. Kids who learn abstinence-only have just as much sex—only they use condoms less often. Limiting the availability of contraception doesn't reduce sexual activity—it just increases unwanted pregnancy. Closing swing clubs doesn't decrease swinging—it just destroys the ongoing community that provides safety, supervision, and dependable social norms.

Some people say that Americans are stupid, that we don't really care about the facts. I believe Americans do care about facts—but we need a context in which to understand these facts. When it becomes clear that the culture wars are not being fought on our behalf to preserve our families, but are being fought *against* us to undermine our expression, health, and choices, Americans will care about the facts.

Today's domestic conservative/fundamentalist political and social movements present a clear (though horrifically distorted) picture of sexuality. It's a narrative of danger and, therefore, of fear; a narrative of sin and, therefore, of self-destructiveness. Erotophobes typically describe their fear in socially acceptable terms: protecting children, supporting marriage, preventing disease, honoring women, sympathizing with the problematic "male sexual psyche."

But they really fear sexuality, *as they understand it*—its awesome power, the temptation to sin, the inevitable destructive decision-making surrounding it, the clear distinction between acceptable activities and unacceptable activities. So they have launched a War on Sex—not just against their own sexuality— against *everyone's*. Their goals are consistent, their strategy coherent. They can frame it in any civic language they want, but it's actually a War on Sex.

As Jeffrey Kuhner, president of the Edmund Burke Institute explains, "Liberals want to create a world without God, and sexual permissiveness is their battering ram. Promoting widespread contraception is essential to forging a pagan society based on consequence-free sex."[1]

The goal of this war is to control sexual expression, colonize sexual imagination, and restrict sexual choices. It seeks to restrict our choices and shape the political/cultural/psychological environment in which we make those choices. It is, at this moment, changing our norms, culture, laws, vocabulary, and our very emotions.

In their never-ending quest to eliminate as much eroticism from American life as possible, erotophobes have enlisted the aid of the largest government in the history of humanity—contemporary American government. Their allies include school boards, zoning commissions, city councils, state legislatures, military leaders, the U.S. Congress, and a series of American presidents. After a near lifetime of self-admitted drinking and sexual carousing, President Bush proudly aligned himself with this side, saying he prays—literally—for a day when those who want to mind their own business (and allow others the same privilege) are conquered by those who want to mind *everyone's* business, imposing their fears and values on the vanquished.

The outcome of these historic battles will determine how our children live—today, and for decades to come. It will determine what books they read in school, what they learn to fear, what private entertainment they're allowed to enjoy, what they know about their bodies, and how much they control their own fertility.

Millions of Americans are afraid of sex. Some admit it, some don't. Millions more hate sex. Again, some admit it, some don't. To deal with their fear and hate, some have declared a war on it. Some admit this, some don't.

If you're interested in sex, you're part of the war whether you like it or not. If you watch TV, use a sex toy, go to the movies, need an abortion, own a Web site, play sex games in bed, use contraception, enjoy spicy online chat, need a physician, or have a child in school, the cannons in the War on Sex are pointed at you.

This book is about that war.

America's pluralism is hated by fundamentalists around the world—including those right here in America. And sexuality is among the last human activities to enjoy the extraordinary, revolutionary promise of American pluralism. So this book is named *America's War on Sex*, not *Congress's War on Sex* or *Newt Gingrich's War on Sex* or *The Catholic War on Sex*. Because America's two centuries of history have been liberating more and more people to drink from the astounding well of democracy. Because it is imperative that we start asking the right questions, right now. And then the answers *will* matter.

And then we'll end the War on Sex.

And the American people will win.

Chapter Two

BATTLEGROUND: SEX EDUCATION—
WHERE CHILDREN COME SECOND

For the children. For the children.

That's the refrain we hear —that their comprehensive efforts to destroy comprehensive sex education are ultimately designed to protect the children.

From sex.

The battle over sex education, however, isn't about what's safe and healthy for the children. It's about what's comfortable (and politically advantageous) for the adults. In the War on Sex, children are cannon fodder. The welfare of our children is being sacrificed so that adults can sleep better at night. It is, of course, supposed to work the other way around.

The battle over sex education comes down to a set of questions about values:

- Should public policy be shaped by science or by belief?
- Should private morality be allowed to shape public education policy? (And if so, what is "moral"?)
- Is childhood and adolescent sexuality a problem to be controlled and suppressed, or a healthy part of life to be understood, celebrated, and shaped?
- Do only children who suppress, avoid, or hide sexual expression deserve protection?
- Do minors have rights to accurate information or health care services?

The battle over sex education is the battle over childhood and adolescent sexuality. The Right and government at all levels have set themselves a clear, if tragic (and ultimately dishonest) challenge: preventing young people from having sexual experiences (and meticulously ignoring their health needs once they do).

They're asking kids to join them in an unholy alliance to deny sexuality—teaching kids to fear sexual feelings, while adults fear sexual information. They've put kids on the front lines of the War on Sex, demanding they patrol a minefield at a crossroads of cultural conflict.

The Bush administration gave the anti-sex educators $1.5 billion, with which they poisoned school children in every state in the U.S. Teaching abstinence has never gone away as a policy priority for the Republican Party, the Religious Right, and therefore many state and local governments. Tragically, abstinence-only-until-marriage is now taught in at least half of U.S. public schools, most private schools, and virtually 100 percent of home-school programs. Probably in your kid's school.

And after a one-year hiatus, federal funding for abstinence has come roaring back.

Meanwhile, regardless of what their parents do or say, the overwhelming majority of today's kids pledging abstinence will have sex before they marry[1]—unless, of course, their parents can magically raise the age of puberty substantially, lower the age of first marriage substantially, dismantle MTV, disconnect the Internet, eliminate cell phones, take over the fashion industry, and reverse 40 years of kids having more privacy because both of their parents (or their friends' parents) work outside the home.

It won't happen.

And so what we're left with is millions of kids being systematically prepared for what they *won't* experience: adolescence and young adulthood without sex. Which means they're being systematically *un*prepared for what they *will* have: sex. Sexual feelings. Sexual relationships. Sexual decision-making.

THE "PROBLEM" OF CHILDHOOD SEXUALITY

Every culture has to deal with the sexuality of its young people. Throughout history, around the globe, boys and girls would typically mate at or near puberty (e.g., Romeo and Juliet). In many cultures, girls and boys are introduced to sex at puberty by older teens, adults, or age peers. Today, the age of consent is 16 or lower in Japan, China, India, and all of Europe except Ireland and Malta.

Most societies around the world have always assumed that young people will be sexual in their early teens, married or not. In some countries, schoolchildren are betrothed to each other and marry in adolescence. In others, schoolgirls are married off as second or third wives to old men. In Africa and elsewhere, clitoridectomy or penile subincision shape youthful sexuality. In Latin America, prostitutes often provide the first sexual experiences for young males (this was common in the United States prior to the 1960s).

But for over a century, America's approach to youthful sexuality has been to minimize, distort, and control sexual knowledge, sexual health, sexual rights, and sexual activity of minors and unmarried young adults. (See, for example, the brutal career of Anthony Comstock.) Today this is achieved in a variety of "modern" ways, such as withholding contraceptive information, supplies, and services; criminalizing consensual teen-teen sex; removing books that mention sexuality from school libraries and school curricula; and forbidding teachers and school counselors from answering certain sexual questions or discussing certain sexual issues.

And through abstinence-only until marriage programs. Unlike other modern countries, America's policymakers don't debate how young to begin teaching kids about contraception, or how to help kids accept their same-gender sexual curiosity, or how young is too young for genital sex, or how to enjoy sex without intercourse. America debates how to most effectively frighten teens and keep them ignorant.

So the main sex education debate in the United States has now degenerated to teaching abstinence versus teaching "abstinence plus." The latter is, "Abstinence is the best and safest form of sexual behavior, but just in case you blow it, here are some important facts you should know." It's as if medical debate were reduced to leeches versus leeches-plus-bloodletting.

Meanwhile, kids still "do it."

They have relationships. They fall in love (regardless of our disdain for their use of the word). They use sex for pleasure or rebellion or revenge. They also use it to discover who they are, what the world is like, and what this amazing thing is that everyone wants so much to keep them away from. Sometimes they want babies. Other times they're giving in to pressure. In other words, they use sex in many ways that adults do.

The original religious injunctions against premarital sex in Western culture were developed when the age of puberty was much higher, and the age of marriage much lower, than they are today (see Figure 2.1). Thus, it referred to a much shorter period in a young male or female's life. And the injunction was about property, not morals. A girl's virginity was considered patriarchal property. If you had sex with a virgin girl, you damaged her father, not her; if caught, you had to compensate him, not her.

With the age of puberty decreasing and the age of first marriage increasing, the average American now spends some 10 years being sexually mature and unmarried.[2] This "premarital sexuality zone" is the largest in human history, and challenges the ideal of virginity-until-marriage in an entirely new way.

Figure 2.1.
Premarital Sexuality Zone

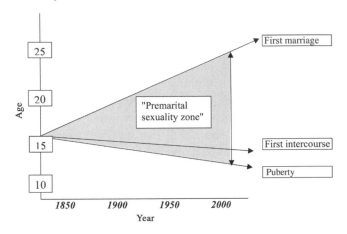

There's never been a generation in human history from whom this many years of abstinence-until-marriage has been expected.

While it's disingenuous to say that we are passive victims of human nature, it is important to know when social policy is attempting to rewrite human history and biology. When abstinence programs talk about traditional family or traditional values, they display their ignorance of how little today's lives have in common with those of even 100 years ago, much less 500 or 1,000.

What are abstinence proponents trying to protect kids from?

- Being interested in sex
- Hearing about various sex practices
- Having sex
- Having sex, resulting in emotional "devastation"
- Having sex, resulting in pregnancy or sexually transmitted diseases
- Breaking God's laws, sinning, or leaving God
- Ruining (or even foreclosing) future marriage
- Liking sex, or getting out of control during sex
- Breaking the female sex role of indifference to sex

Every one of these is a nightmare for those who war on sex. These fears explain why the premarital sexuality zone is a problem zone. At least in this regard, these people take sexuality seriously. They see sex as the ultimate gateway drug.

SOLUTION: WHAT IS "ABSTINENCE EDUCATION"?

In the 1970s, American policy aimed to reduce teen pregnancy (and the resulting teen births). It was the golden age of comprehensive sexuality education: contraceptive decision-making, communication skills, values clarification.

But that changed in 1981. A year after completing his tenure with the Christian Broadcasting System (as a consultant to founder Pat Robertson), Senator Jeremiah Denton (R-AL) proposed to stop teen sex with the Adolescent Family Life Act. It would fund school and community programs "to promote self-discipline and other prudent approaches" to adolescent sex. It was dubbed chastity education.[3] This pointless Victorian exercise has been operating ever since—with a gigantic budget Senator Denton couldn't have dreamed of. It was, and is, the answer for everyone afraid of teen sexuality: abstinence-until-marriage.

While much of the abstinence movement is sneaky, they are honest about one thing: their goal is to indoctrinate a whole generation (and, of course, each succeeding generation). They want to change the culture of young people about sexuality, away from it being a means of self-expression, a way to get touching, a source of personal power (for better or worse, of course), a form of self-exploration and relationship rehearsal, and a vehicle for actual intimacy. Instead, they want kids to fear sex as something dangerous, something seductive that leads to shame, pain, and a ruined future. Somehow, this is all supposed to change on their wedding night. Pioneer sex educator Sol Gordon described this message as "sex is dirty—save it for someone you love."[4]

The abstinence project is no less than transforming desire and eroticism from a semi-familiar, normal part of life to a not-understood, estranged enemy.

Different programs define abstinence differently. While a few say that non-intercourse sex is OK, others exclude any non-genital sex, and some even exclude any activity (such as dancing or masturbating) that generates sexual thoughts or ideas. Regardless of definition, every abstinence program says it's for the children. No one admits it has anything to do with decreasing adult anxiety.

Abstinence education is the substitution of restriction for thinking and decision-making. As shown in Figure 2.2, it substitutes an abstinence zone for the premarital sex zone. It's a zone that has been getting bigger every decade for the past century.

Abstinence education could be designed to be honest and dignified. (It could even be made more effective; see Taverner and Montfort, *Making Sense of Abstinence* [2005]). But in today's America, abstinence training is none of these. It is so wrapped up in lies, inaccuracies, and values presented as f acts that it is hard to respect the message. And as presently designed, it is impossible for kids to get value from these programs without paying an enormous price.

The Federal Definition for Abstinence-Only Programs

The term "abstinence education" indicates an educational or motivational program with *all* of the following features:

- Has as its exclusive purpose teaching the social, psychological, and health gains to be realized by abstaining from sexual activity
- Teaches abstinence from sexual activity outside marriage as the expected standard for all school-age children
- Teaches that abstinence from sexual activity is the only certain way to avoid out-of-wedlock pregnancy, sexually transmitted diseases, and other associated health problems
- Teaches that a mutually faithful monogamous relationship in the context of marriage is the expected standard of sexual activity
- *Teaches that sexual activity outside of the context of marriage is likely to have harmful psychological and physical effects. Teaches that bearing children out-of-wedlock is likely to have harmful consequences for the child, the child's parents, and society*
- Teaches young people how to reject sexual advances and how alcohol and drug use increase vulnerability to sexual advances
- Teaches the importance of attaining self-sufficiency before engaging in sexual activity

Also, note that if any contraceptive method is discussed, its "failure rate" must be mentioned, *not* its "success rate." The only exception is the failure rate of abstinence, which is *never* discussed.

Section 510(b) of Title V of the Social Security Act, P.L. 104–193

Let's say society were to systematically withhold other vital information from kids—say, how to take care of their teeth. Toothpaste and floss would become illegal, the need to brush daily hushed up, the effectiveness of braces lied about, teens taught that gum disease can be prevented only by not eating sushi.

Or say that Congress decided it didn't want certain kids (maybe the children of immigrants, or New Yorkers, or Mormons) to do well in school. We'd see widespread disinformation about study habits, libraries secretly relocated, bibliographies discredited as unreliable, and kids told that completing their assignments on time might hurt their eyes.

How would America react? Wouldn't there be editorials and non-profit organizations standing up for those kids at risk for lifelong oral pain and school failure? How long could such policies endure?

Figure 2.2.
Abstinence Expectation Zone

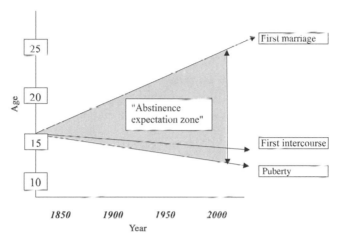

BENEFITING ADULTS, NOT KIDS

The war on sex education pretends to be about kids' needs, and proponents say they want to protect kids from disease, pregnancy, and broken hearts. But abstinence programs don't protect kids from disease, pregnancy, or broken hearts. That's because they aren't effective at postponing sexual involvement or at making kids safer when they do have sex. For example, a Florida State University evaluation study found that after taking an abstinence-only program, kids were more likely to agree that they *should not* have sex before marriage than before they began the program. But over the same period, their sexual behaviors *increased.*[5] And most abstinence programs assume kids aren't already having sex—which would be pretty funny if it weren't so dangerous.

So abstinence programs don't help kids. But they do benefit adults—both emotionally and financially. Abstinence programs help adults convince themselves that kids are less sexual than they really are. They get to maintain the illusion that kids aren't doing it, are going to stop doing it, or aren't going to start.

These programs also allow parents to believe that they don't have to have a long series of talks about sex over a period of years. If kids aren't having sex, and all they need is to be told, "Don't do it," there's no reason to discuss it more than once or twice. Abstinence programs encourage parents to evade one of their key responsibilities.

And abstinence programs allow adults to feel that their kids are safe from sin, hell, and religious error (and from unauthorized pleasure). For parents who believe in such things, this concern is an enormous burden. Relief from this concern is worth almost any price to them. In this case, that price is hurting the kids about whom they're so concerned. Abstinence also relieves their anxiety about kids' autonomy and personal power, a key religious concern.

At the very least, the clear message kids learn from abstinence programs is, "If you have sex, *do not tell us*. We will be disappointed in you, God will hate you, everything around here will change." Many adults crave the relief that their kids' deception provides. They make kids responsible for reducing adult anxiety about childhood sexuality. But this means that as soon as kids have sex, they lose the special relationship with their parents that they may need more than ever.

The ubiquity of the abstinence goal and its programs has been a turning point in the War on Sex, both politically and financially. Abstinence has brought the War on Sex into everyone's living room. Even if you're not kinky, don't want to go to a swing club, don't want an abortion, don't look at porn or strippers, and don't even have cable TV, if you have kids, abstinence brings the War on Sex into your home. If you believe in pluralistic democracy—even if you're religiously inclined—it's arguably the single biggest challenge to your values as an American and as a sexual person.

Abstinence programs are also a forum for an explicit anti-gay agenda, although that can hardly be part of helping heterosexual kids be abstinent. (As a bonus, they terrify the millions of average heterosexual kids who think about, or experiment with, same-gender sex.) They validate adult delusions about human nature—that fear is the best motivator of behavior, that sexual decision-making is simple, that young adults can routinely abstain from sex into their mid-twenties (when most Americans marry).

IF IT DOESN'T WORK, WHY PROMOTE ABSTINENCE? FOLLOW THE MONEY

The other major impact of abstinence is its economic windfall for (already tax-exempt) churches and faith-based organizations. Through it, individual churches, after-school programs, and so-called pregnancy crisis centers (actually anti-abortion centers) have received hundreds of millions of dollars—more support than received by all the people displaced by Hurricane Katrina or all the people with handicaps in the United States.

As Leslee Unruh, founder of the National Abstinence Clearinghouse, has noted, "Abstinence has become a business," one which Unruh estimates has increased by more than 900 programs in recent years.[6] Abstinence has been a monster growth industry (see Figure 2.3).

The abstinence industry is a huge federal and state gravy train, but only for a narrow segment of Americans. Because *non-abstinence* sexuality programs—scientifically based programs that counsel kids to make good sexual decisions,

Figure 2.3.
Federal Funding for Abstinence-only Programs

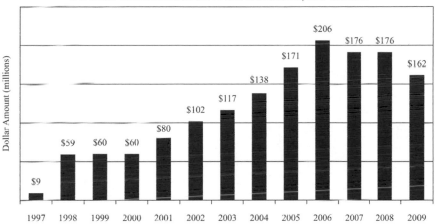

TOTAL U.S. ABSTINENCE FUNDING, BY YEAR

to use contraception when they decide to have intercourse, to appreciate non-intercourse sex, to discuss sex with their parents, to develop good communication skills, to learn more about their bodies—*are not eligible* for this money. This is government money strictly for ideologically correct groups. Groups, of course, that vote. Abstinence programs are a new and completely legal way that the federal and state governments funnel hundreds of millions of dollars to religious groups that support them politically.

These funds, of course, find their way to those with political connections. The Best Friends Foundation received $1.5 million between 2003 and 2004; it's run by Elayne Bennett, wife of William Bennett, and Alma Powell, wife of Colin Powell. The Medical Institute of Austin, Texas, has received more than $500,000 annually; its founder, Joe McIlhaney, has been friends with George W. Bush since he was governor. And (disgraced) former House Majority Leader Tom DeLay's (R-TX) congressional district has received almost a half million dollars in funding annually.[7]

Your money is being used to persuade your kid to not start having sex or to stop having sex, and, either way, to feel bad and to mistrust contraception and disease protection. Your money. Your money.

As the icing on the cake, recipients of these hundreds of millions were never required to prove that their efforts are effective. More on that later.

THE STRUCTURE OF AMERICAN "ABSTINENCE"

In one sense, the policy goal of abstinence-only education is simple enough: persuade young people to not have sex *before marriage*, no matter when that is (and if you're not legally allowed to marry, tough). To do this, their strategies include:

- Persuade young people that contraception and disease protection are so unreliable that they must not be trusted.
- Persuade young people that premarital sex always has dreadful consequences.
- Provide young people various forums for publicly committing to abstinence.

The first strategy requires lying. Because condoms work. They work better today than they ever have. They work so well, hundreds of millions of people around the world use them to shape when and if they'll have children. They work so well, virtually every sero-discordant couple (one partner is HIV positive, the other HIV negative) who use condoms regularly prevent the HIV negative partner from contracting HIV.[8] They work so well, they help prevent herpes, chlamydia, and the newest STD demon of the Right, HPV. In the 1980s, they helped dramatically stem the tide of HIV among gay men.[9]

Contrast this with these lies told by the Abstinence Clearinghouse:

- "Condoms provide 0 percent protection against HPV."
- "Condoms do not protect against . . . genital herpes."
- "Trusting a condom to protect your health puts your future at risk."
- "Trusting condoms . . . is like playing with fire. Sooner or later you get burned."[10]

The second strategy relies on presenting belief or opinion as fact—which also constitutes lying. A common lie of abstinence, for example, is that premarital sex ruins future marriage. But where's the data? Abstinence advocates trot out depressed Susie in Omaha and dysfunctional Pedro in Denver, and yes, of course those anecdotes are true. But they aren't representative. And what about kids who become terrified of sex due to abstinence programs? Girls who learn that boys only want one thing? Boys who learn to feel guilty for masturbating? Abstinence programs have no data about any of this.

Abstinence programs should be honest: "We don't think anyone should have sex before marriage because it's wrong. Period." But they don't trust the power of their own values-laden message. They bolster their message by lying about the consequences of premarital sex: depression, suicide, poor marriage options, isolation, damaged health.

The third part of the abstinence strategy is providing forums for abstinence commitment. Public ceremonies, Ring Thing, virginity pledges, and so forth sound good, and it's easy to assume that kids are sincere when they do it.

But the idea that 14-year-olds can make commitments that they will honor when they are 19 is ludicrous. Again, there's no data to support this theory of human development. In fact, 88 percent of teens pledging abstinence have sex before marriage—that is, abstinence *fails*. And it fails at a dramatically higher rate than condoms or any other contraceptive method—even unreliable methods like withdrawal or rhythm.[11]

Public virginity pledge forums are always religiously oriented. For example, the Silver Ring Thing's parent organization says it is an "evangelistic ministry" by which it is bringing "our world to Christ." Young people who attend and pledge virginity until marriage receive an "Abstinence Study Bible" and purchase a silver ring inscribed with a reference to the Bible verse, "God wants you to be holy, so you should keep clear of all sexual sin." Participants are also encouraged to accept Christ as their savior.[12]

In response to an ACLU lawsuit, federal funding for the Silver Ring Thing was grudgingly suspended in August 2005. Consequently, the Silver Ring Thing was required to restructure its program to be non-religious in order to continue to receive federal funds. But its homepage says it "promotes the message of abstinence until marriage centered in a relationship with Jesus Christ." As founder Denny Pattyn tells teen audiences, "Unless you have God right here [patting his heart], at the center of this decision, I think you'll struggle keeping this decision [holding up his ring finger] of putting on a ring."[13]

As usual with sexuality, the Right wants it two ways. They want to claim sex is bad for kids and abstaining is good; when confronted with the data challenging this, they say, well, abstaining is good morality. OK, then it's a moral position—which people can differ over. Then they say that, well, all our kids deserve protection.

Kids using abstinence *this weekend* will have sex. They've promised they won't, but they will. How do we want to prepare them for this? We tell kids to wear seat belts, even though we don't want them to crash. We tell kids to call if they'll be late, even though we want them home on time.

What do we offer kids who don't refuse sex the way we want them to? Nothing—no backup plan, no mnemonic devices, no support, no information to protect themselves. Ask an abstinence proponent what a kid should do if he or she has sex, and they reply, "Don't have sex." Denny Pattyn, founder of Silver Ring Thing, says that if "my own 16-year-old daughter tells me she's going to be sexually active, I would *not* tell her to use a condom."[14]

Abstinence "educators" disregard kids who have sex like so much trash. It's a disgusting form of hostility toward our young people. It would be like withholding vitamins from kids who refuse to eat vegetables (after promising they will), or withholding toothbrushes from kids who drink soda (after promising they won't).

Abstinence: How Government Subsidizes Religion

Most of the $1 billion that promoted abstinence-only-before-marriage from 1997-2008 was awarded to agencies over which there was no program oversight whatsoever. A huge amount of this taxpayer money went to religious organizations—which all Republicans wanting to be president in 2012 say they wish to resume.

Here are just a few examples:

Pennsylvania

Catholic Social Services	$46,000
Lutheran Social Ministries	$231,000
St. Luke's Health Network	$92,000
Shepherd's Maternity House	$50,000
Silver Ring Thing	$400,000

California

Catholic Charities of California	$361,605

New York

Catholic Charities of New York	$2,500,000

Illinois

Roseland Christian Ministries	$800,000
Lawndale Christian Health Center	$461,278

SO WHAT'S IN THEM?

After just a few years of dramatically increased funding, both anecdotes and advertising made it clear that abstinence programs were more ideology than education.

In 2002, Congressmember Lois Capps (D-CA) offered an amendment to a congressional funding bill that would have required abstinence programs receiving federal money to be scientifically accurate. Nothing fancy—just be accurate.

But the amendment was soundly defeated—it was simply too much to ask that our kids' health would be handled with facts rather than beliefs. Such "accuracy amendments" were introduced in many subsequent years, including a 2006 amendment with 120 congressional cosponsors. The result was always the same: abstinence proponents—politicians, religious figures, civic leaders—said, "Whose science?" as if they could actually provide competing data showing that abortion does lead to infertility, premarital sex does lead to suicide, gays are mentally defective, or condoms do fail to protect against disease.

In 2004, Congressmember Henry Waxman (D-CA) released a report, "The Content of Federally Funded Abstinence-Only Education Programs." It's a concise evaluation of the 13 most popular abstinence-only sex education programs.[15] It documents that "over 80 percent of the abstinence-only curricula used by 2/3 of [federally funded programs] contain false, misleading, or distorted information about reproductive health." Especially common were:

- False information about the effectiveness of contraception
- False information about the risk of abortion
- Blurring religion and science
- Treating stereotypes of girls and boys as scientific fact
- Scientific errors

Here are actual quotes from these federally funded programs that actual children in actual American schools are still reading and hearing:

- "In heterosexual sex, condoms fail to prevent HIV approximately 31 percent of the time"
- "Touching another person's genitals 'can result in pregnancy.'"
- "The popular claim that condoms help prevent the spread of STDs is not supported by the data."
- "Women gauge their happiness and judge their success by their relationships. Men's happiness and success hinge on their accomplishments."[16]
- "Following abortion, according to some studies, women are more prone to suicide."
- "Personal problems 'can be eliminated by being abstinent until marriage.'"

The Religious Right's response (e.g., Morality in Media, Focus on the Family, Agape Press) was predictable: they trashed Waxman. They linked him to same-sex marriage. They attacked him for quoting Planned Parenthood data. They criticized his acceptance of campaign contributions from "groups that financially benefit from abortion" like the American Medical Association. They complained that he didn't mention all the existing funding for safer sex programs.[17]

Since they say they care about kids, you'd imagine they were concerned, wanting to fix the programs, increase their ability to serve kids, enhance their credibility, and so forth. Instead, they attacked the report, the congressional representative, his district, and his supporters. They attacked science.

No programs attempted to improve themselves. No one apologized for or attempted to remove inaccuracies. This is clear proof that these programs are far less interested in their results than in their ideological purity—and their hundreds of millions of dollars in funding.

EVALUATION? JUST SAY NO

Abstinence programs resisted outside evaluation from the very start (at the same time that political conservatives were demanding that public schools and teachers prove their effectiveness). Abstinence leaders didn't want their programs evaluated for three reasons: (1) they believed so earnestly in the ideology of the programs that they didn't care about the actual impact, (2) they valued the adult anxiety reduction provided by the programs, (3) and they didn't want any negative data to jeopardize the government wealth flowing their way.

For years, when confronted with questions of effectiveness, the motto of abstinence programs was "Just say, 'I don't know.'" An evaluation requirement was never built into these programs. They got away with this for years.

Then–Senate Majority Leader Bill Frist was particularly hypocritical about this, as he proudly strutted his support of health care outcomes research. In 2000, he said that outcomes research was a priority "of federal efforts to improve the quality of health care in the United States."[18] And in 2003, he said, "We must continue to move forward in the collection and the evaluation, dissemination, and analysis of information related to everyday health care."[19] But the outcome data on sex education programs already existed, *and he promoted federal policies contraindicated by the data.*

Program evaluation is a sophisticated science used by trained experts across the industrial world, including the United States. It *is* possible to know how abstinence programs affect both thinking and behavior in its recipients— if someone wants the facts. Proponents of comprehensive sexuality education have wanted to know for decades, and so there are peer-reviewed, validated, and replicated studies about their programs. In reality, science has now conclusively shown:

- Does sex education make kids have sex?
  No
- Do condoms work?
  Yes
- Does the availability of condoms in school clinics increase kids' sexual activity?
  No

- Does premarital sex itself lead to problems?
  No
- Does abortion lead to breast cancer?
  No
- Do abstinence programs stop kids from having sex before marriage?
  No

The biggest lie about abstinence is that it works every time. It *doesn't*. In the most comprehensive study ever done on adolescent health and sexuality, Columbia University's Dr. Peter Bearman's investigators interviewed more than 20,000 young people about virginity pledges. Twelve percent of the students who pledged virginity kept their promise. That's a 12 percent success rate with this supposedly perfect method. That means abstinence fails 88 percent of the time—*six times as often as condoms fail in typical use*, six times as often as the method that abstinence advocates say is unreliable.[20]

In 2007, a 164-page report was published evaluating the actual results of participating in abstinence programs. The federally funded report ("The Mathematica Report") documented clear findings, including:

> Youth in the [abstinence] program group were no more likely than control group youth to have abstained from sex; among those who reported having had sex, they had similar numbers of sexual partners and had initiated sex at the same mean age.[21]

The study was so well done it received the 2009 Outstanding Evaluation Award from the nonpartisan American Evaluation Association (AEA), which praised the nine-year study "for its rigor, balance, and impact, which led to major changes in federal policy and funding." For one glorious moment, it looked like we might actually be getting rid of abstinence.

CONSEQUENCES OF ABSTINENCE EDUCATION

So take a billion dollars, create a bunch of religious and ideological programs filled with inaccuracies, provide no oversight, and after a few years, what do you get? Before Columbia's study, before Mathematica's study, information was already trickling out: *These programs don't work*. Here are just a few of the many local and peer-reviewed studies that were done:

- In Minnesota, sexual activity of junior high school participants in an abstinence program doubled.[22]
- Young people who took a virginity pledge are one-third *less likely* than non-pledgers to use contraception when they become sexually active.[23]

- Young people who took a virginity pledge have the same rates of STDs as non-pledgers.[24]
- Teens who pledge abstinence and haven't had intercourse are *more likely* to have oral and anal sex than non-pledgers who haven't had intercourse.[25]
- Two-thirds of Northern Kentucky University students who pledged celibacy until marriage broke that pledge while still in college. Of those who remained "abstinent," more than half acknowledged having oral sex while describing themselves as celibate.[26]

Did you know this? Probably not. It should be front page news—"Billion-dollar program crucial to saving youth of America *doesn't work*."

Predictably, America inherited the consequences of the failure of all three abstinence strategies (lie about safer sex, claim that beliefs are facts, and provide forums for abstinence pledges). Kids don't abstain—whether they think sex is dangerous or not; whether they make public pledges or not; whether they think God will be mad at them or not. Over 90 percent of Americans have sex before marriage. The only question is whether they will have it in a physically and emotionally healthy environment. The goal of abstinence programs is to ensure they *won't*.[27]

Although the emotionally abusive messages of abstinence programs don't shape adolescents' sexual *behavior* in their hoped-for ways, they do shape the *emotional context* of adolescents' sexual behavior. So these young people use contraception less, understand less about how sex actually works, feel worse about themselves, and talk less about their sexual feelings or experiences with their parents. So abstinence programs create the worst of both worlds: non-abstinence, lower rates of contraception and disease protection, and less intelligence about sex—not only logistically, but emotionally and spiritually.

All this from people who say they care about the children.

Without question, many young people would be better off if they postponed sex by a year or two or more. (Of course, many adults would, too.)

But no social policy is cost-free. And every public policy has unexpected consequences—some of them quite unpleasant. So what do kids pay for abstinence programs?

- Unfamiliarity with, and mistrust of, contraception
- Increased contraceptive risk-taking
- Reinforcement of the belief that sex is bad and dangerous
- Reinforcement of traditional gender roles
- Unrealistic expectations of marital sex
- Unrealistic expectations of their virgin-until-marriage future
- Ignorance of appropriate, personal sexual decision-making

- Shame, guilt, and isolation when chastity vows are broken
- Healthy experimentation made complicated and more dangerous
- Feeling rejected and judged by parents and/or God

Abstinence advocates say that a comprehensive (they call it "mixed") message teaches kids that we expect them to fail. That assumes, of course, that shunning sex is the only form of "success."

But what does it do to young people when we actually do set them up to fail? We are training a whole generation that when they have sex before marriage, they will have failed, that God will be angry, that they lack discipline or self-respect or love for their future partner. They will also learn that they can't plan effectively. What kind of parents, citizens, lovers will they then be? With how many bad feelings will they associate sex—thereby undermining thoughtful sexual decision-making?

Abstinence training is a huge gamble—if kids "fail," they can't protect themselves. So even if a few kids benefit, the rest—the majority—pay the price. Is this a reasonable social policy—gambling that a few will make it and abandoning the rest?

And as award-wining educator Bill Taverner asks, how are programs preparing young people to make the transition from using abstinence to using a different method of contraception and disease prevention? Even if abstinence programs do help teens postpone sexual involvement, morality—yes, morality—dictates that kids be prepared for the time when they will switch to a different way of life, with different challenges. So long as abstinence programs ignore this reality, their claims of "morality-based sex education" are hollow.

A PAUSE IN THE ABSTINENCE TRAVESTY—BUT ONLY A PAUSE

Comprehensive sex education programs did pop up periodically in a few places. And as unnecessary and life-damaging teen pregnancies continued to sadden and outrage parents, a few local school districts and legislators bravely tried alternatives to abstinence. But despite the fact that they'd been scientifically tested, such programs were typically attacked.

For example, not all Wisconsin schools currently have sex education. But the state's Healthy Youth Act passed in March 2010 required schools that do teach sex education to teach students medically accurate, age-appropriate information, including how to use birth control and prevent STDs. Parents, of course, could excuse their children from sex-education classes.

Within a month, Juneau County District Attorney Scott Southworth notified the county's five school districts, saying the new law promotes sexual assault of children, and warning that teachers who follow the law could be charged with delinquency of a minor, with punishment of up to six years in prison.

"For example," Southworth wrote, "if a teacher instructs any student aged 16 or younger how to utilize contraceptives under circumstances where the teacher knows the child is engaging in sexual activity with another child—or even where the 'natural and probable consequences' of the teacher's instruction is to cause that child to engage in sexual intercourse with a child—that teacher can be charged under this statue. Moreover, the teacher could be charged with this crime even if the child does not actually engage in the criminal behavior."

Southworth's letter encouraged recipients to share it with school boards in their communities in an effort to get them to end sex education programs rather than follow the new state mandate.[28] (See later in this chapter for the ironic update.)

And in August 2011, a Catholic parish in Rochester, New York, joined with a local "crisis pregnancy center" to mobilize opposition to the new condom availability (and expanded teen health courses) in the nurse's office of city high schools. This, despite an opt-out option for parents who do not want their kids to have access to those condoms.[29]

This kind of ignorance and prejudice is common across the country, political embers waiting to burst into flame the moment a Republican or conservative is in power—not just in the White House, but in the State House, school boards, County Commissions, and local legislatures.

It's for the kids.

BACK TO ABSTINENCE—AS QUICKLY AS POSSIBLE

In October 2011, House Republicans released their 2012 spending bill. Among other devastating cuts to vital health and education programs, the bill slashed funding for medically accurate programs to reduce teen pregnancy, from $105 million to $20 million. In addition to cutting the funding, the legislation removed the requirement that funded programs be supported by rigorous research or promising models—the requirement on which the programs' effectiveness was based.

As a sadistic bonus, the legislation completely eliminates funding for Title X, the nation's family planning program.

"House Appropriations Committee Chair Hal Rogers (R-KY) and Subcommittee Chair Denny Rehberg (R-MT) should be ashamed of themselves for perpetrating such deficit-reduction hypocrisy and continuing the Republican assault on sexual and reproductive health," said Monica Rodriguez, President and CEO of Sexuality Information and Education Council of the United States (SIECUS).[30]

As the 2012 presidential campaign gets rolling, Republicans and "conservative" Democrats are polishing their anti-sex, anti-teen credentials promoting abstinence. Organizations like CharlestonTeaParty.org and the National Abstinence Education Association are circling the campaign like hyena, just waiting to move in for the federal abstinence dollars they anticipate will be available after the election.

State legislatures are also getting into this anti-science, faux morality act: in 2011, for example, Wisconsin's Senate passed a bill that would require school sex education to promote marriage and abstinence as the best way to prevent pregnancy and sexually transmitted diseases.

KIDS AS A MINORITY TARGETED FOR DISCRIMINATION

When it comes to sexuality, Americans under 18 are a repressed minority. In most or all states:

- Information is systematically withheld from them
- Government, school, and church programs deliberately lie to them
- Health services are withheld from them
- Health products are withheld from them
- It is against the law for them to take photos *of themselves* in provocative poses
- In many states, it is against the law for them to have intercourse with *anyone*

In other arenas, kids have rights, regardless of the needs and feelings of adults. There are laws, for example, requiring school attendance and certain vaccinations, and restricting child labor and corporal punishment, regardless of how parents or other adults feel about these issues.

But when it comes to sex, young people have no rights. Not *insufficient* sexual rights—virtually *no rights*. Their rights have been taken away in response to adults' hysteria about their safety, anxiety about their morality, anger about their autonomy, confusion about their decision-making, and rejection of their human needs.

Sure, we regulate kids' access to tobacco, alcohol, and driving. But there's science backing these decisions, and kids are allowed access to unlimited, accurate *information* about these subjects. And we rarely tell them that young people who smoke or drink (or have car accidents) are bad, selfish, and immoral, no matter how much we want to discourage them.

Not so regarding sex.

When the United States has treated other minority groups similarly (Native Americans, people with handicaps, women, etc.), scandal has eventually ensued, and discrimination has decreased. There is still no real public scandal about the way America targets children and young adults for discriminatory treatment.

International human rights law establishes that every person, including every child, has the right to the highest attainable standard of health; the right to seek, receive, and impart information of all kinds; the right to non-discrimination and equal protection of the law; and the right to an education.[31] This includes the right to information and education concerning the prevention and control of prevailing health problems.[32]

The United States has signed international treaties guaranteeing these rights, including the International Covenant on Civil and Political Rights,[33] the International Covenant on Economic, Social, and Cultural Rights, and the Convention on the Rights of the Child. Participating countries affirm their legal obligation to refrain from "censoring, withholding or intentionally misrepresenting health-related information, including sexual education information." The U.S. has clearly not met this basic standard.

The 1998 United Nations guidelines on HIV/AIDS and human rights recommend that nations "ensure that children and adolescents have adequate access to confidential sexual and reproductive health services, including HIV/AIDS information, counseling, testing and prevention measures such as condoms."[34]

But according to the 2002 report of the internationally respected Human Rights Watch, "[American] federally funded abstinence-only programs, in keeping with their federal mandate, deny children basic information that could protect them from HIV/AIDS infection . . . these programs not only interfere with fundamental rights to information, to health and to equal protection under the law. They also place children at unnecessary risk of HIV infection and premature death."[35]

Children as collateral damage in America's War on Sex? That would be bad enough. But the repulsive truth is that, in this war, children are a primary target.

Chapter Three

THE MOST POWERFUL "MINORITY" IN THE UNITED STATES

The new Helms School of Government at Liberty University ... [will] train young people to enter public service with a Christian worldview and a bold passion to confront a liberal-oriented culture. Students will spend weekends and summers working hand-in-hand with pastors and staff members of evangelical churches all over America, registering voters in the churches and neighborhoods along with educating parishioners.

—*Jerry Falwell*[1]

I'm confused. Exactly who is this "they" that the Religious Right keeps saying has hijacked the country?

The Religious Right keeps bragging about how they are responsible for electing the Congress (and elected the last president, and will elect the next). They take credit for getting many conservative federal judges appointed. They claim they are electing mayors, state legislators, and governors across the country. So who exactly is passing the laws we all live under?

And who are the consumers of the cultural products the Religious Right constantly criticizes? Who do they think is watching *Desperate Housewives*, going to see *Maid in Manhattan*, buying *Cosmopolitan*, and downloading Janet Jackson's half-second of nipple? At the mall, who do they think is giving their 13-year-olds money to buy belly shirts, iPods, and cell phones?

America's most popular recreations include NASCAR races, TV wrestling, and poker. All involve beer and half-undressed pretty girls. Fans for these events are disproportionately from blue, conservative, religious states.

And pornography: The Right keeps complaining that we're "flooded" with it. Yes, there are 50 million Americans consuming porn—and they aren't all Al Gore and Michael Moore. So who are these 50 million people? When the Right complains that hotels are making a fortune selling in-room porn, who do they think stays in those hotel rooms in Topeka, Provo, and Memphis?

The Religious Right has masterfully portrayed itself as the voice of the sex-sober majority being oppressed by the sex-crazed minority. They demand sympathy and righteous indignation about the way "children," "families," "tradition," "morals," "values," and "decency" are under attack. They have gotten the government and media to support them as defenders of America's wholesomeness—against some mythical, incredibly powerful (and immoral) "them."

But the Right is like the kid who kills his parents and asks for mercy because he's an orphan. Somehow, they neglect to mention that it's the consumer choices and other preferences of *their own constituents* that are the so-called problem. It is average, working-class and middle-class Republican voters in Charleston, Abilene, and Spokane who are watching porn, having affairs, buying vibrators, going to strip clubs, and keeping *Sex and the City* on the air. People may tell pollsters and even politicians that they want more "decent" programs and products. But that's not what these people are discussing, buying, and watching. Religious people, conservative people, "decent" people demand, and get, *Gilmore Girls*, a Hitachi magic wand, Kim Kardashian, Jenna Jameson, a lap dance.

The Right portrays America as under siege by a dangerous ideology, a villainous intelligence, which simply doesn't exist. But not only isn't it evil, it isn't *out there*. It's the ordinary, everyday decision-making *of its own people*. And they make the same choices people around the world make whenever they have a chance.

Unfortunately, the idea of a tangible satanic force that must be battled out in the world is familiar to tens of millions of fundamentalist and evangelical Christians. At various times, the group said to embody this Evil has been identified as pagans, Jews, Muslims, Catholics, Mormons, and communists. These days they're homosexuals, liberals, and pornographers.

To the Right, these three symbolize choice. Valuing pleasure. The rejection of fear of Evil. A loss of group control over individual impulse.

The Religious Right plays to the literalist expectation of Evil exquisitely; for example, look at its portrayal of less than civilized, less than adult, conscienceless, seductive homosexuals. Somehow, this group of six or seven million people, with no guns, two congressmen, and Ellen DeGeneres, is positioned as a threat to the most powerful country in the history of the world. This narrative is a brilliant political accomplishment.

What exactly *is* this "homosexual agenda" from which the Christian Right is protecting you and me? The idea that same-gender marriage hurts "traditional" marriage is staggeringly silly. "Honey, I'm sorry I had an affair, but you know how those gays are undermining our marriages ..." Our government has cut funding for student loans, alternative fuels research, grandma's medication, poor people's birth control, and job retraining. But the Christian Right says the real danger we face is a bunch of men and women who want to marry each other instead of, uh, each other.

WEAK AND BULLIED? HARDLY

Here are just four recent ways in which organized religion, far from being marginalized by a godless culture, actually has a central seat at the table of political power and policy making.

Pulpit Freedom Sunday

Since it's legal to participate in religion, and legal to participate in politics, inevitably some people do both. As long as this is done on a personal level, the Republic is not endangered: Go ahead and believe in the Rapture (a more common American belief than Evolution) and vote for Joe or Sam. No problem.

There is, however, the issue of taxes—billions of dollars of taxes. The IRS exempts approved churches from paying taxes. The income of church-owned operations— from bakeries, parking lots, hotels, farms, and so on—is over $150 billion annually (that's way more than the budget of the entire state of California). In exchange for this exemption, the government asks for two things:

1. A little bit of paperwork.
2. Don't preach politics.

For this, many religious leaders and followers feel persecuted. On top of this multi-billion-dollar giveaway, they demand the right to influence elections organizationally. Remember, every member of a church is free to vote as she or he wishes, to contribute money to candidates, to write letters to newspapers and congressmembers.

On the annual Pulpit Freedom Sunday (next scheduled for October 7, 2012), pastors across the country are encouraged to explicitly endorse candidates from their pulpits during church services. This civil disobedience is designed to goad the IRS into challenging some church's tax-exempt status; the idea is that this enforcement will be so unpopular that the federal law barring electioneering from the pulpit will be overturned.

"Contrary to the misunderstandings of many, tax-exempt status is not a 'gift' or 'subsidy' bestowed by the government," according to the Alliance Defense Fund and its senior legal counsel, Erik Stanley.[2]

This clearly demonstrates mainstream religion's sense of entitlement rather than its marginalization. The Church believes it is owed tax exemptions worth billions of dollars *and* the right to elect candidates. And the political issues on which The Church demands to speak? Not poverty, not air pollution, not mass transit: reproductive rights, sex education, adult entertainment, the rights of sexual minorities, contraception. See a pattern?

They demand to participate in the highest possible way in America's War on Sex.

Texas Constitution Demands Religious Belief

... nor shall anyone be excluded from holding office on account of his religious sentiments, *provided he acknowledge the existence of a Supreme Being.*
—*Texas Constitution, Article 1, Section 4*

Says Deana Pollard, law professor at Texas Southern University's Thurgood Marshall School of Law, "In this case, we do have a constitution that's unconstitutional."[3]

Concerned Women for America—In Bed with Virginia's Politicians

Concerned Women for America (CWA) claims to be the country's largest public policy women's organization. Their mission is "bringing Biblical principles into all levels of public policy, focusing on six core issues: the family, the sanctity of human life, religious liberty, education, pornography and national sovereignty."[4]

In the world real, that translates to criminalizing abortion, eliminating comprehensive sex education, censoring pornography, reducing church-state separation, and eliminating all adult entertainment. Apart from their retro interest in "national sovereignty," this is the exact agenda of the War On Sex—by "bringing Biblical principles into public policy."

So how are they doing this? Consider one of their typical fundraisers, held May 26, 2011. Hosted by Virginia's attorney general, the event is a troubling mix of the state's political and religious power elite. The invited guests included the governor, lieutenant governor, secretary of state, and congress-members, not to mention various candidates for elected office. CWA doesn't hide its religious agenda at all; the bottom of the invitation features a quote from Corinthians.[5]

Carving out Special Religious Law

In 2005, the Constitution Restoration Act was introduced in both the House and Senate. A pet project of those advancing Dominionism, it would have limited the power of the federal judiciary specifically in religious liberty cases. The bill also stated that judges or other court officials who listen to cases that meet these criteria are to be impeached and convicted. Just what America needs—more divisive exemptions for religious issues from the laws of our country.

"The acknowledgment of God is not a legitimate subject of review by federal courts," says one of the bill's authors—Roy Moore, the same judge who lost his job for putting religion above the law (see Chapter 13).

* * *

The Right is correct about one thing. The American family and American community are, today, spinning out of control. But it isn't because of the Axis of Moral Evil—homosexuals, liberals, and pornographers. Rather, it's the unintended consequence of a wildly advanced capitalist system, which gives spending money and privacy to teens, while sending jobs overseas, over-working two parents who can't afford health care, geographically dispersing families, and increasing our grandparents' life spans while decreasing their dignity. It's a socio-political-economic system that values computer network-ing over intimate connecting.

Our alienation and sense of powerlessness is the unfortunate result of get-ting what Americans said we wanted—more and better gadgets with which to avoid reality, more low-density housing in car-dependent suburbs, more guarantees of physical security, and more certainty about the most uncertain anxieties of human existence—no matter how deadening our jobs, how unhealthy our environment, how corrupt our politics, how meaningless our entertainment, or how atomized our families and relationships. Americans have asked for lives that require less thinking, and we've been handed them. At a soul-searing price.

We ought to be sympathetic about the fear, grief, and resentment of people watching their lives and communities spinning out of control, and their kids spinning away from them. Men and women across America are broken-hearted. And the primary political group addressing this heartbreak is the

Religious Right. Unfortunately, they do it in a fundamentally disempowering way. They say, "Let's give in to our fear, let's restrict our choices and disown our rights, let's attempt to control everything and everyone *else*." Sexuality—messy, idiosyncratic, unpredictable, transgressive—is high on the agenda of what needs controlling.

They don't encourage us to grow up and face our own role in creating lives we fear and resent. But as the only political group discussing heartbreak and isolation, they attract listeners, listeners who become disciples. And so although Christians damn the very activities the public values—soft-core entertainment, hard-core stimulation—the public somehow feels comforted. When the Right talks about an idealized, wholesome past that never existed, that's code for wanting to address how frightened and lonely people feel now. That makes people feel acknowledged. They then want to say "yes" to whatever solution is proposed, even the loss of dignity, freedom, and adulthood that is the core of the Religious Right's program.

So when the Religious Right hyperventilates, sputters, rages, and prophesies doom regarding premarital sex, extramarital sex, non-marital sex, and pornography, abortion, *Grey's Anatomy*, STDs, and dildos, they're talking about themselves but blaming a "them." People who feel powerless are cheering this war on "them," even though it's ultimately a war on *themselves*. But people who feel powerless and ashamed of their own sexuality can't possibly stand up for themselves in this battle. They will continue to cheer Sarah Palin, Rick Santorum, Sam Brownback, James Dobson, Richard Land, and Brent Bozell as they demonize porn and Fox TV—even while voters buy porn and watch Fox. And manipulated by these cynical leaders, the same voters will continue to spit on the American Civil Liberties Union while it protects their rights to buy porn and watch Fox.

There's a good chance that the Christian Right will continue scoring serious victories. They actually could criminalize abortion, restrict porn, abolish strip clubs, eliminate gay adoptions, purge and re-closet homosexuals, and make adultery and premarital sex excruciatingly frightening and costly.

But no government and no religion can eliminate the desire for sex, for sexual experimentation, for the taboo, the naughty, the novel, the intense. See the most recent century of Western civilization. Read the last century of science fiction: No matter how dystopian the fictional society, no one can stop people from somehow creating erotic entertainment and pleasure *outside* the bounds of whatever is considered "decent."

We know that many notable figures on the Right—including Rudy Giuliani, Jimmy Swaggart, Bill O'Reilly, Strom Thurmond, Robert Livingston, David Vitter, Laura Schlessinger, John Ensign, Carl Paladino, Arnold Schwarzenegger, Mark Sanford, and Newt Gingrich—have participated in extramarital affairs, visits with prostitutes, and sexual harassment. Who would *they say* is the "them" who's hijacking the country?

Chapter Four

BATTLEGROUND: REPRODUCTIVE RIGHTS

"I would like to outlaw contraception. It is disgusting—people using each other for pleasure," says Joseph Scheidler, national director of the Pro-Life Action League. Some people are obsessed with the "rights" of sperm to fertilize eggs, and with fertilized eggs to implant. Operation Rescue founder Randall Terry says, "I don't think Christians should use birth control." In fact, some in the anti-choice movement have attacked fellow activists for not opposing contraception. As University of Dallas Professor Janet Smith says, "It is foolish for pro-lifers to think they can avoid the issue of contraception and sexual irresponsibility and be successful in the fight against abortion."[1]

Clearly, their logic is backward: Obviously, the way to eliminate abortion is to eliminate unwanted pregnancy. They should ardently *support* birth control, but they don't. Aspiring presidential candidate Rick Santorum says he cannot support availability of the Pill. During a Senate debate intended to minimize contraceptive coverage by insurance plans several years ago, Senator Dick Durbin (D-IL) said, "I was stunned when I came to Congress many years ago to find that the people most vehemently opposed to abortion were equally opposed to contraception. How can that make sense?"[2]

WHY REPRODUCTIVE RIGHTS?

Other than your partner, and possibly your mother, why would anyone—especially a stranger—care about whether you use a condom, keep emergency contraception (EC) on hand, or have an abortion?

It starts with a belief that the only legitimate purposes of sex are reproduction and marital intimacy. Contraception symbolizes sex for other purposes—that is, pleasure. Thus, an attack on contraception is an attack on sex-for-pleasure. And that's what the battle over reproductive rights is all about—limiting sex for pleasure.

So forget "pro-life." Forget "birth control pills cause cancer." Forget "condoms don't protect against a broken heart." Listen to what else the anti-sex "conservatives" are saying:

- "When people are less afraid of sex, they have it more."
- "Birth control causes promiscuity."
- "People need to understand that their actions have consequences."
- "God doesn't want anyone using birth control or getting an abortion."

These are not public health messages. They are the strategic thinking of people trying to control the amount and type of sex that *everyone* has.

Why *everyone*? After all, if you think abortion is horrible, don't get one. If you think an IUD or diaphragm dehumanizes you, don't use one.

While many Americans believe that whatever two adults do privately is their own private affair, many others disagree. For them, sex is either authorized or unauthorized. And sex is authorized only between legally married heterosexual couples, generally limited to penis-vagina intercourse. The only legitimate reasons for this sex are reproduction and, according to some clergy, strengthening the bond of holy matrimony.[3] This means that most Americans are having unauthorized sex. Put another way, most of the sex people have in America is unauthorized, including the sex had by most religious conservatives.[4]

Those who war on contraception and abortion don't just want to discourage everyone from having unauthorized sex. They want to prevent it, or at least make it as difficult as possible. They may call themselves pro-life, but they're really anti-choice. Anti *your* choice.

Why do these people want all unauthorized sex to stop?

They feel it pollutes their world. Obsessed by unauthorized sex, they feel it degrades everyone, even those not participating in it. They don't seem to have the psychological tools to ignore what others do behind closed doors.

Because they are attempting to adhere to a very rigid sexual standard, temptation appears everywhere. Understandably, they fear their own (generally rather ordinary) sexual impulses, which they project onto others. Fearing their own sexual decision-making, they mistrust others'. They even talk about "slippery slopes"—that if you think you can "get away" with, say, premarital or extramarital sex, there's no limit to what else you'll do.

Ultimately, they characterize sexuality as dirty, and therefore incompatible with spirituality, which they claim is what drives them—and legitimizes their attack on your rights.

American government at the national, state, and local levels has created public policy to discourage unauthorized sex and minimize contraceptive use. This itself is a breathtakingly radical development. The policy isn't quite perfectly sealed yet: You can still buy condoms in Safeway (although astonishingly, Safeway can't freely advertise them); most single Americans do have sex (although getting birth control pills and EC is becoming harder for them); and abortion is only legal and accessible for *some* people *some* of the time (if you aren't a teenager, are less than 3 months pregnant, can afford to travel several times, can find and afford a provider, and can stomach the lectures or sonograms you're forced to endure). But these current parameters aren't the point.

The point is that our government has decided to care about what you do sexually. Again. This time it isn't what you do with your eyes, mouth, or imagination, it's what you do with your genitalia. Your federal and state governments care about what you do with your genitalia way more than they care about what you do with your arms or legs. And they aren't even honest about the reasons. So let's examine them.

FEMALE EMPOWERMENT

Here's another reason some people want to limit or eliminate everyone's access to contraception and abortion: These technologies enable women to transcend the limited role of mother. Studies from around the world show that such movement is the gateway to more financial and psychological independence.[5]

Reproductive knowledge and practice has always been part of female folk culture. Birth control techniques have been practiced in virtually all societies, including herbal potions, ritual infanticide, abortion, magic, withdrawal, vaginal inserts, douches, and cervical caps.

The nineteenth-century legal bans against abortion and contraception were introduced partly to eliminate midwives (seen as competition by increasingly professionalizing doctors), and partly to undermine women's emerging reproductive control. And America's industrialization and westward expansion led government and religious groups to desire population growth. In 1905, President Theodore Roosevelt attacked birth control and the new trend toward smaller families as decadent, a sign of moral disease—and a dangerous response to the huge influx of immigrants who were "weakening" America's gene pool.

Fifty years later, the new contraceptive technologies of the mid- and late twentieth century were seen as particularly progressive because they could potentially sever the link between sexuality and reproduction. Shulamith Firestone emphasized this would free women from the "tyranny of reproduction," which dictated women's oppression.[6]

These technical advances were opposed by conservative and religious forces on so-called moral grounds. But their hypocrisy was exposed a few years later. Whereas abortion and contraception *challenged* the traditional equation of femininity and motherhood, radical new fertility technologies helped *fulfill* the traditional female role—and were therefore approved by most Christians. Artificial ways of *enabling* reproduction were OK, whereas artificial ways of *preventing* it were not.[7]

As one book put it, "The use of birth control requires a [social] morality that permits the separation of sexual intercourse from procreation, and is related to the extent to which women are valued for roles other than wife and mother."[8] But only a few years after the Pill and *Roe v. Wade*, it was no longer just contraception that was believed to disrupt the natural connection between mother and conception or fetus, it was the new kinds of artificially aided fertility, with human eggs and embryos moving in and out of a woman's body, or even from one woman's body to another. Sperm was being geographically manipulated as well.

Whether surgical, biomedical, or pharmaceutical, who will have access to any new technology, and under what circumstances?[9] Some attempt to frame this as a moral or spiritual or health question, but it's most properly seen as a *political* question. Perhaps this is more obvious if the question is posed as, "Who shall be allowed to access the Internet in North Korea?" "Who may have a GPS locator in China?" "Which adults shall be allowed to drive a car in Saudi Arabia?"

SEVERAL STRATEGIES

The war on reproductive rights is carried out in several ways at once. The strategies are:

1. Increasing the unwanted consequences of unauthorized sex.
2. Decreasing the motivation for using some or all kinds of contraception and abortion.
3. Limiting access to contraceptive and abortion equipment, technology, and information.

The churches, civic groups, and government agencies that promulgate these policies and restrict our choices uniformly claim that they care primarily about the disadvantages of various contraceptive/abortion technologies and the personal consequences of their use. And these days, some believe that abortion is morally wrong.

But this is disingenuous. None of the disastrous results they say they're trying to protect us from are actually supported by science. For example, the idea that abortion leads to depression, infertility, and breast cancer, or that premarital sex leads to depression and suicide, are simply untrue. Scary, but *not true. They are as untrue as the idea that the sun revolves around the Earth.*

Besides, don't Americans deserve the chance to evaluate the costs and benefits of their own choices—and aren't we used to doing so? For example, some people feel flying in planes is dangerous, and so they don't, while others think its benefits make flying an acceptable risk. The same is true with driving on New Year's Eve, smoking cigarettes, getting a facelift, and enlisting in the Marines.

Here's how your reproductive rights are being *successfully* challenged.

INCREASING THE UNWANTED CONSEQUENCES OF UNAUTHORIZED SEX

Those who war on sex depend on a simplistic hypothesis repeatedly proven wrong throughout history: that if you increase the risks and dangers of sexual expression, people will stop having sex. This shows such a dramatic lack of insight into their fellow creatures, one could be forgiven for imagining they had never met another human. Fear of AIDS has not prevented Africans from having sex, the risk of capital punishment has not prevented Iranian gays from having sex, and the possibility of unwanted pregnancy has not prevented millions of American teens from having sex.

And yet the fear (no statistics, just fear) of your "promiscuity" is routinely cited as justification for public policy. Examples include withholding access to contraception for teens, and the cancellation of condom distribution in American prisons.

This was the idea the government and Christian conservatives trotted out in attempting to restrict your access to emergency contraception (the "morning after pill" or EC). They said they feared that the drug would lower the risks of sex, thereby encouraging you to have more sex with more partners.

Discouraging such behavior is a function of the family (and church), *not* the government. Besides, studies show that access to the drug does *not* increase contraceptive risk taking.[10] Unfortunately, this *fact* (and very positive safety data) has not influenced the anti-sex movement's desire to discourage access to and use of the drug (for details about the government's campaign against EC, see "Exiling Emergency Contraception" sidebar, pp. 40–41).

The latest twist in this irrational saga is the development of a vaccine that can *prevent* HPV—the Right's favorite STD, because it can lead to cervical cancer. To be effective, the vaccine must be administered *before* a girl becomes sexually active. Remember, the Right is always pointing to HPV/cervical cancer as a tragedy people should avoid by abstaining from unauthorized sex.[11] Then it attacks this medical marvel by claiming, without any data whatsoever, that the vaccine will increase "promiscuity" by reducing the possible consequences of sex. ("That's OK, Kevin, I'm vaccinated so I can't get HPV, which can lead to cervical cancer. Come on inside me!") Thus, they're against *anyone* using it.[12]

And what's their alternate strategy for unmarried women to avoid getting HPV when they have sex? Unmarried women shouldn't have sex. This clearly illustrates that they are far less interested in supporting people's health than they are in controlling our sexual behavior. Their intellectual dishonesty is spectacular.

DECREASING THE MOTIVATION FOR USING CONTRACEPTION AND ABORTION

Although reliable contraception is a modern marvel, waging war on sex requires undermining people's motivation for using these products and procedures.

Contraceptive information is, of course, systematically withheld from sex education in most American schools—often by explicit requirement. Any young person who develops the habit of using contraception to prevent unwanted pregnancy will have to do so in spite of what he or she learns in school. (For more information, see Chapter 2.)

Anti-sex forces continue to lie about the effectiveness of condoms. After years of urging condom use to prevent HIV, the Centers for Disease Control and Prevention's (CDC) Web site started doubting their efficacy in 2005, until a firestorm of criticism forced a resumption of scientific information. The following year, the Food and Drug Administration (FDA) proposed requiring labels on condom packages that warn that they are probably less effective against certain STDs, including herpes and HPV, than others.[13] President George W. Bush had been lobbying for such condom labeling for years.[14]

It isn't only the American government that is willing to lie about condoms to discourage their use. For years, James Dobson (Focus on the Family), Jan LaRue (Concerned Women for America), and many others have been talking about how condoms don't protect people very well. The Catholic Church's continuing stance against condoms as being somehow "immoral" extends to its opposition to using them to prevent AIDS. In 2003, the Vatican stirred international controversy with its false claim that the HIV virus can pass through condoms.[15]

Popes on AIDS

In 2005, Pope John Paul II reaffirmed church teaching urging abstinence and marital fidelity to stop the spread of AIDS—and forbidding condoms. As *New York Times* columnist Nicholas Kristof commented, "The worst sex scandal in the Catholic Church doesn't involve predatory priests. Rather, it involves the Vatican's hostility to condoms, which is creating more AIDS orphans every day. The Vatican's ban on condoms has cost many hundreds of thousands of lives from AIDS. Historians . . . will count its anti-condom campaign as among its most tragic mistakes in its history."[a]

In 2009, Pope Benedict XVI reignited the controversy over the Catholic Church's position on condom use. As he made his first trip to Africa, the Pope said condoms were not the answer to the continent's fight against HIV and AIDS—in fact, that condoms could make the problem worse. The timing of his remarks outraged health agencies trying to halt the spread of HIV and AIDS in sub-Saharan Africa, where an estimated 22 million people are infected.[b]

Following an international meeting about preventing and treating AIDS in 2011, Monsignor Zygmunt Zimowski, head of the Pontifical Council for Health Care Workers, attempted damage control by citing Pope John Paul II on the "crisis of values" behind the AIDS epidemic. Church officials said Pope Benedict believes that condoms are an ineffective tool for preventing AIDS (which contradicts all known research), and that they promote "immoral behavior."[c]

The Catholic Church operates a lot of clinics, hospices, and other programs for people with AIDS worldwide, especially in Africa, the continent hardest hit by the disease. But Church-run programs cannot distribute condoms as long as the Pope condemns them, and can only tout the Vatican's position against them.

[a]Nicholas D. Kristof, "The Pope and AIDs," *The New York Times*, May 8, 2005, http://select .nytimes.com/search/restricted/article?res=F10A14FD3E540C7B8CDDAC0894DD404482.
[b]http://www.guardian.co.uk/world/2009/mar/17/pope-africa-condoms-aids.
[c]http://latino.foxnews.com/latino/health/2011/05/30/popes-hiv-condom-view-helpful-unaids -tells-vatican/.

ABORTION: LEGAL BUT INCREASINGLY PUNITIVE

The Right attempts to discourage women from getting legal abortions by making the process so difficult or repulsive that many women just give up. Increasingly, individual states are using techniques such as mandatory waiting periods, forced exposure to photos or ultrasounds, and mandatory, propaganda-filled lectures.[16]

Exiling Emergency Contraception

Wouldn't it be great to have a product that could minimize one of the worst heritages of rape and incest; help prevent families from self-destructing; give foolish or unfortunate young people a second chance at a mature, responsible future; and in general, reduce the problematic consequences of sexual intercourse?

There is such a product: emergency contraception (EC). Essentially a high dose of conventional birth control pills, it has been available in Europe and the United States for decades. It prevents pregnancy for up to 72 hours after intercourse. That's the window—72 hours. The common side effects are uncomfortable, but nothing outside of any woman's ordinary experience, and certainly absolutely nothing compared to an unwanted pregnancy.

Despite religious and civic group opposition, the FDA finally approved EC for prescription use in 1999. Obviously, though, a person needing it needs it immediately, so it must be available over-the-counter (OTC) and kept on hand. Although there's absolutely no rational reason it shouldn't be, a few key government officials and religious leaders successfully prevented all of America from having this access.

Faced with an application to make EC available OTC, the FDA first cited bogus safety issues. Then it created a long series of unexplained delays. When Director of the FDA's Office of Women's Health Susan Wood resigned in frustration, and several senators demanded an explanation, the government and religious establishment finally admitted their objection: easier availability of EC would cause "promiscuity."

For example, Dr. David Hager, one of only four FDA committee members who voted against OTC availability, said, "What we heard today was frequently about individuals who did not want to take responsibility for their actions, and wanted a medication to relieve those consequences." And Tony Perkins of the Family Research Council said that making EC available OTC "would make the morning-after pill the new Saturday night party favor of choice."[a] Americans' response should have been simple and direct—"So what?"

Concerned Women for America has trashed the drug, saying it "can lead to promiscuity; it's for the promiscuity lobby." By which, presumably, they mean those people lined up demanding that young people ruin their lives.[b]

Those ranting that EC leads to "promiscuity"—a life of depravity which is, of course, every American's God-given right—have clearly failed to read the boring social science literature that shows conclusively that EC *doesn't* increase "promiscuity."[c] Of course the literature is irrelevant to religious zealots who don't trust science. They don't trust sex, and they don't trust you.

In September 2005, Senator Orrin Hatch (R-UT) called it not "a pharmaceutical issue as much as it's a social issue."[d] Although most people nodded in agreement, this is a staggering admission for a modern democratic nation. What exactly *is* the social issue? It's the technological reduction of the risks of sexual activity, challenged by the desperate desire to maintain those risks.

In November 2005, the non-partisan Government Accountability Office confirmed that the FDA's decision process denying EC's OTC availability was "unusual," and cited evidence of uncharacteristic high-level participation and obstruction. A decision about America's health had become completely politicized—a politics obsessed with fundamentalist Christian "morality."

Susan Wood, who had resigned as head of the FDA's Office of Women's Health in protest, said she was "very worried" that political pressure from the same conservative groups who had blocked OTC for EC would also delay availability of a new vaccine that protects against HPV, and therefore against cervical cancer. And for the same reason—that reducing one of the risks involved in sexual contact could lead to "promiscuity" among young women. As we've already seen, she turned out to be absolutely right. "I also worry when and if we reach an HIV vaccine," she said, "that they will raise the same argument."[e] Of course they will—increasing the risks of sexual activity is their stated mission.

[a]http://www.motherjones.com/news/update/2005/11/planb_timeline.html
[b]http://www.cwfa.org/articledisplay.asp?id=7967&department=CWA&categoryid=life
[c]Reproductive Health Technologies Project, at http://www.rhtp.org/news/media/documents/Factsheet-ThecaseforOTCPlanBAug05.doc
[d]New York Times, 9/2/05
[e]http://www.alertnet.org/thenews/newsdesk/N16618935.htm.

In 2011, 80 state measures were enacted that restrict access to reproductive health care.[17] Thirty-four states *require* that women receive *scripted* "counseling" before receiving an abortion, something not required prior to far more dangerous procedures such as plastic surgery or heart bypass surgery. South Dakota requires that a woman be informed that abortion "will terminate the life of a whole, separate, unique, living human being" with whom the woman has "an existing relationship." Six states require disclosure of a false[18] link between abortion and breast cancer. Three others require information on possible psychological impacts of abortion, including straightforward lies[19] about suicide and depression. In 2005, three states introduced bills that would require patients to view ultrasounds of their fetus, or "unborn child," as South Dakota wants to require.[20]

Twenty-four states currently *require* a waiting period (typically 24 hours) between counseling and abortion. This necessitates two separate trips to a clinic, an enormous burden for poor women or those responsible for children—especially in states where women have to travel hundreds of miles to get to an abortion provider. Since the passage of Mississippi's mandatory counseling and waiting period law, abortion rates have fallen, the number of women going out of state for an abortion has risen, and *the proportion of second-trimester abortions has increased.*[21]

Mandatory counseling "ignores women's First Amendment rights to decline to attend anti-abortion lectures," says Wendy Kaminer at the Atlantic.[22] "Think about a similar law that would require pregnant women, or women planning pregnancies, to undergo counseling about the risks of childbirth, the economic costs of raising children, and the possibility that they'll break your heart."

Ten states now require women be told that the fetus may feel pain during abortion, and three require anesthesia be offered directly to the fetus. In 2005, bills were introduced in Colorado and West Virginia that would *require* fetal anesthesia *regardless* of a patient's consent or additional risk.[23]

Kansas now provides grants to organizations that encourage women to carry their pregnancies to term, and prohibits grants to groups that provide abortion. Minnesota has appropriated $5 million to encourage women to carry their pregnancies to term.[24]

ABORTION TRAINING AND AVAILABILITY

The number of abortion providers in the United States fell from 2,400 in 1992 to 1,793 in 2008,[25] while our population increased by 50 million. Meanwhile,

- In 2008, 87 percent of all counties in the United States lacked an abortion provider; 35 percent of all American women aged 15 to 44 live in those counties.[26]
- Only 11 percent of all abortion providers offer abortions at or beyond 24 weeks.[27]
- One out of every four women must travel more than 50 miles to obtain an abortion.[28]
- Three states have only *one* abortion provider.

At the same time, fewer and fewer medical residents are receiving training in reproductive health services. Only 20 percent of the nation's OB-GYN residency programs require first- and second-trimester abortion training. More than a third of chief residents in family practice receive no training to fit a cervical cap, fit a diaphragm, or insert an IUD. In Maryland, 97 percent of family practice residents and 36 percent of OB-GYN residents had no experience in elective termination of pregnancy in the first trimester. Of their family practice residents, half had never inserted an IUD, 43 percent had never inserted an implant, over a third had never prescribed emergency contraceptive pills, 30 percent had never fitted a diaphragm, 90 percent had never fitted a cervical cap, and 83 percent had no experience with tubal sterilization.

CATHOLIC HOSPITALS

The Catholic Church continues to buy hospitals across the United States, and these Catholic hospitals are now the nation's largest single group of non-profit medical facilities. The Catholic Church operates over 600 hospitals and 1,400 nursing homes, hospices, and clinics, and dozens of health care systems.[29]

These institutions provide some of America's finest health care. Their beliefs and regulations about sexuality, however, conflict with the needs of tens of millions of patients. The National Conference of Bishops' "Ethical and Religious Directives for Catholic Health Care Services" unambiguously *forbids*:

- Abortion
- Providing contraceptive information and devices
- Issuing or providing information on EC
- Voluntary sterilization
- Disseminating AIDS and other STD information involving condoms

According to data collected from 597 of these Catholic-run hospitals, only 5 percent of them provided EC on request. An additional 23 percent will provide EC to rape victims, but typically with onerous conditions, which can include pregnancy testing, proving they were raped, and police intervention.[30] Over half of Catholic hospitals refuse to offer EC to patients under *any* circumstances, including rape.[31] And only half of the hospitals that don't offer EC give ER patients a referral elsewhere for EC.[32]

The refusal of these hospitals to provide normal health care services is particularly onerous as Catholic hospitals buy up secular facilities across America. Of the 127 mergers involving church-run and secular facilities between 1990 and 1998, nearly half resulted in the immediate termination of some or all reproductive services. For example, a Poughkeepsie, New York, hospital ended abortion services after merging with a Catholic hospital, and a Gilroy,

California, hospital ended sterilization and contraceptive services after such a merger. As fewer institutions offer reproductive health care, the elimination of a single facility can add hours or even days to the task of getting legitimate services.[33]

Health care at Catholic colleges is similarly compromised. Of 133 Catholic colleges responding to a 2002 survey, only 16 made contraceptives available to students.[34] In 2011, the Association of Catholic Colleges and Universities fought to exempt its members from new federal health care regulations requiring the provision of contraceptive services for students and employees—many of whom are *not* Catholic.[35]

Half of the Church's 600 hospitals are funded by taxpayers—who have a variety of religious beliefs (including 34 million who claim no religion). If Catholic hospitals can accept money from the government, they should be required to provide the standard professional services offered by American medicine. Of course, no patient who rejects sexual health care services is forced to accept them—which should make this simple. Only the politics of religious exceptionalism allows Catholic hospitals to be exempt from the normal rules regulating other government-funded hospitals.

FETAL RIGHTS LEGISLATION— AND WORSE, "PERSONHOOD"

Fetal rights measures have been introduced in every state. They grant a fetus the same rights guaranteed to people in state constitutions. This is critical not only in criminalizing abortion should *Roe v. Wade* be overturned. It will also figure in battles over the *definition* of abortion. For example, some legislators, pharmacists, and religious crusaders are calling EC, which *prevents* pregnancy, an abortion drug. If a fetus has significant legal rights, a legislature could outlaw EC on the grounds that it *may* harm the fetus. Indeed, a Michigan lawmaker has introduced a bill to ban over-the-counter sales of EC in his state in case the FDA legalizes it.[36]

In 2004, Congress enacted the Unborn Victims of Violence Act, which calls a fetus a "child in utero" and defines it as a legal victim if he or she is injured or killed during the commission of a federal crime of violence. Thirty-eight states now have "feticide" laws, defining the killing of a pregnant woman as killing two "people." This language was conspicuous in California's highly publicized 2004 Scott Peterson "double murder" (Laci Peterson was pregnant) trial.[37]

Legal recognition of fetuses' rights is *not* the same thing as criminalizing abortion—it's *worse*. Nor is it the same as declaring when life begins. It's more pervasive, with a cascade of awful, medieval effects. This is not an incremental change, it is an earth-shaking event counter to every founding document and principle in American history. In essence, law has enshrined beliefs—not facts, beliefs—into legal entities. Law has taken moral and metaphysical beliefs and made them facts.

This *can't* be done without compromising the rights of women, whose bodies keep fetuses alive. Mothers are always free to not get abortions, always free to treat their fetuses as if they have legal standing—say, by leaving them money in a will. *But giving a fetus legal standing diminishes the rights of the mother in whose body it's growing.* This is a radical step that places an unfair burden on any pregnant woman (and her partner and any other children she has).

As the Feminist Women's Health Center says, "The life of a fetus cannot be separated from the life of the pregnant woman. [Doing so] is unique in medicine and law. No one can create a set of medical or legal principles giving a right to life to the fetus, because doing so inevitably limits the woman's rights."[38]

And this is no abstraction. Various states are now arresting and even jailing pregnant women for behavior deemed detrimental to their fetuses. The National Advocates for Pregnant Women had to file a federal civil rights challenge to a South Carolina hospital policy of searching pregnant women for evidence of drug use (and giving the information to police).[39] Some 300 women have been arrested in South Carolina alone for fetal endangerment.[40]

The anti-choice movement clearly cares far more for fetuses than for babies, although babies are *at least* as human as fetuses, thus deserving equal protection. But controlling how people treat already-born babies doesn't help the religious community in their project of controlling sexuality. So we should not be surprised that Mississippi has the most stringent restrictions on abortion in the country *and* the highest infant-mortality rate. So much for the moral, "pro-life" culture of which they are so proud.

The "personhood" movement is even more draconian than fetal rights legislation. This movement would give a fertilized egg rights *before* implantation—which is the way "pregnancy" has been defined for a century. These people actually claim their definition is based on scientific fact, when of course it's just an arbitrary opinion. After all, many, many fertilized eggs *don't* implant, get flushed out of the body, and no one's the wiser. Shall we mourn each of these?

According to PersonhoodUSA, "The science of fetology in 1973 was not able to prove, as it can now, that a fully human and unique individual exists at the moment of fertilization."[41] A fertilized egg is "fully human"? What exactly does that mean?

"The key to defeating Roe v Wade is Personhood," their Web site says. They're right, of course.

Held Prisoner in a Hospital Because Her Fetus Had "Rights"

In 2009, Samantha Burton was held prisoner in a Florida hospital because she was pregnant, and her fetus had "rights."

Burton was 25 weeks pregnant in March 2009 when she showed signs of premature labor. At her obstetrician's urging, she sought care at Tallahassee Memorial Hospital. Found not to be in labor, she was told to remain on bed rest.

When Burton tried to leave the hospital to get a second opinion, her obstetrician refused to let her go, and then obtained a county court order requiring Burton to undergo "any and all medical treatments" that her physician, acting in the interests of the fetus, deemed necessary. The Court held the hearing by telephone; Burton had to argue her case from her hospital bed without an attorney or independent medical opinion. Three days into her court-ordered confinement, Burton underwent an emergency C-section, at which time the fetus was found to be dead.

With the ACLU's assistance, Burton sued. The hospital argued that it had a duty to protect the fetus under Florida's child welfare statutes. The ACLU noted that this was a dangerous precedent: "To ignore this fundamental constitutional distinction between the state interest in protecting fetal life and its interest in protecting the lives and health of people is to risk virtually unfettered intrusion into the lives of pregnant women."[a]

On August 12, 2010, the Florida Circuit Court of Appeals found in favor of Burton and against the State.[b]

"When you see these cases," says Lynn Paltrow, executive director of the National Alliance of Pregnant Women, "It makes me think we're still engaged with a fundamental question of whether, upon becoming pregnant, women are still full citizens."[c]

[a]http://www.salon.com/2010/01/14/forced_bedrest/.
[b]http://en.wikipedia.org/wiki/Burton_v._Florida.
[c]http://www.thedailybeast.com/newsweek/2010/01/18/the-prenatal-problem.html.

EXAMPLE: INVENTING THE RIGHT TO REFUSE

In response to the legalization of abortion in 1973, federal and state policymakers started enacting "refusal clauses." These laws allowed doctors to refuse to perform or assist in abortions, and hospitals to refuse to allow abortions on their premises. It was a creative and effective way to circumvent the new law.[42]

Since then, refusal clauses have spread to an ever-expanding group of work-ers and activities—always involving sex. A few years ago, for example, a Wis-consin pharmacist refused to fill, *and actually confiscated*, a single woman's prescription for birth control pills. An Illinois ambulance worker refused to transport a patient suffering severe abdominal pain to a clinic for an emer-gency abortion. Now some hospital workers are refusing to clean surgical instruments or handle paperwork they believe are tied to abortion.[43]

Medical facilities in every state can now refuse to provide abortions. This creates huge obstacles for women who can't afford (or aren't healthy enough) to travel the hundreds of miles now sometimes necessary, not to mention the problem of follow-up care. Many states now protect any institution that refuses to *mention* EC to women who have been raped.

In Nebraska, The Nebraska Catholic Conference demands that all mental health professionals maintain the right to refuse to treat any client because of reli-gious or moral convictions. Social workers are fighting to insist that the Depart-ment of Health and Human Services at least require counselors who refuse to help gay clients *to refer them to professionals who will*. The Nebraska Catholic Conference, in a clear statement of its lack of human empathy, is resisting.[44]

In 2010, when enacting health care reform legislation, Congress continued existing religious exemptions from professionalism and ethics by granting refusal rights to the newly formed exchanges—including the right to refuse to refer or give factual information. State laws continue to protect *any* health care employee who refuses to participate in even the most indirect administration of a procedure to which he or she objects "morally"; in states such as Mississippi, payers of health care are allowed to refuse to cover any service to which they object on moral grounds, which could include steriliza-tion, HIV treatment, STD diagnosis or treatment, contraception, or even prenatal checkups for women who "shouldn't" be pregnant.[45]

"Moral grounds." Today, that's code for *sex*. "Morality" hasn't led pharma-cists to demand the right to refuse to fill prescriptions for drugs tested on ani-mals, or drugs whose manufacture pollutes the environment, or drugs that are too expensive for anyone but the wealthy or well-insured, or drugs with awful side effects, or drugs that make children violent or adults submissive zombies. No, "moral grounds" invariably means, "Makes sex safer or more enjoyable."

Shockingly, most states now allow pharmacists to refuse to fill any legal pre-scription, and to refuse to refer patients to other pharmacies that will help them. The American Pharmacists Association wants to protect "pharmacists' rights to not dispense drugs they are opposed to." The Christian Legal Society's Center for Law and Religious Freedom says it's un-American to ask pharmacists to sac-rifice their rights for their jobs. The Family Research Council wants the Work-place Religious Freedom Act passed to protect pharmacists' rights to uphold their "morals" at work.

Compromising Professional Training: How "Moral" Is That?

On October 5, 2011, the Michigan House of Representatives introduced House Bill 5040, which gives students in mental health training programs the right to refuse service to any client because of a "sincerely held religious belief or a moral conviction."

This means students being trained as psychologists, social workers, and marriage counselors will not be required to learn how to deal with any discomfort, judgment, or prejudice in a clinical setting. Students will not be expected to grow, nor to learn about any cultures, family structures, or sexual practices of which they disapprove. While this proposed law is framed as honoring the "rights" of students, it is a way of institutionalizing prejudice and social disapproval. It is a guarantee that people involved in alternative lifestyles, people who are atheists, and people needing assistance using contraception or abortion (among others) will have less access to quality counseling than others. It will also invite some students to demonstrate their piety (to self as well as others) by refusing to work with a larger and larger group of clients.

Pharmacists do not have this "right." Your Aunt Mabel does—*in private.* Indeed, pharmacists have the same rights as your Aunt Mabel to withhold, cajole, persuade, and bully in order to shape your behavior—in private.

Pharmacists and pharmacies are licensed by the state to provide health care. As such, they must adhere to standard U.S. medical practices and serve the entire community, regardless of race, ethnicity, age, height, eye color, and shoe size. Or medication requested, or condition it's designed to treat. That's the responsibility pharmacists take on in exchange for the privileges of their license. Anyone is free to believe that some people should not have access to certain medications—but acting on this belief disqualifies a person from being a pharmacist.

Imagine a psychotherapist who believes that the state law prohibiting him from having sex with patients conflicts with his sincere moral beliefs. Would we give him federal protection when he sleeps with his patients?

Discrimination is discrimination, whether a pharmacist bases it on *your* religion or *hers.* Refusing to sell medication to help an unmarried woman have responsible sex is just as bad as refusing to sell a black family a house in a white neighborhood. Or should people's religious beliefs allow them to do this, too?

Enforcing "Morality" on Others

Shall there be any limit on people's right to enforce their morality on others? If pharmacists demand this right, what about other people demanding their rights? These might include:

- A cab driver refusing to take you to a Planned Parenthood clinic
- A 7-Eleven clerk who won't sell you alcohol because you shouldn't drink
- A Bloomingdale's clerk who won't let you spend any money on goods made in China
- A toy store clerk who won't let you buy toy guns or sexy Barbies
- A physician who won't let you have a blood transfusion that's against God's will
- A lawyer who won't write a will leaving your money to your lazy son
- A high school counselor who won't help a girl get into MIT because girls shouldn't be scientists

Since some pharmacists demand the right to withhold any medication that facilitates sex-related behavior of which they disapprove, we can also expect to hear the following rationales for being refused legally prescribed medication:

- "No, that estrogen for your sex-reassignment interferes with God's creation of men and women."
- "No, you're gay, and you'll use that Viagra to have abominable gay sex."
- "No, treating your vaginal infection will allow you to resume sex— which, since you're single, you shouldn't be having."
- "No, that medication will relieve the pain of a vasectomy you shouldn't have had."
- "No, antidepressants will make you a more feisty woman, disrupting family harmony."
- "No, Prozac will make it hard for you to ejaculate, indirectly limiting your family size."
- "No, testosterone will increase your postmenopausal sex drive, and there's no need for that."

The government's job is to set standards based on science so that consumers, who can't possibly evaluate professional competence, are safe. Consumers can then use any criteria they like, including moral values, to decide which medications and procedures to use or avoid. *That's* the American promise.

The Bible, while silent on abortion, repeatedly demands humility and compassion. Pharmacists who won't dispense EC to a woman who has only a few hours left to prevent an unwanted pregnancy need to have their Viagra prescription denied, their blood pressure medication delayed, and their eyeglass prescription confiscated. Since their religion hasn't taught them compassion, perhaps these experiences would.

Chapter Five

THE SEXUAL DISASTER INDUSTRY

There is so much money to be made scaring the hell out of Americans about sexuality that no one on this gravy train can afford to slow it down. Any outsider who questions this juggernaut is immediately labeled insensitive, anti-family, immoral, or a pedophile.

The Sexual Disaster Industry (SDI) involves federal and local government, conservative religion, so-called morality organizations, right-wing think tanks, victim-parade daytime talk shows like *Maury* and *Dr. Phil*, and news programs looking for a bump ("Isn't it awful the way people go to strip clubs? Film at 11!"). Honorable mention goes to the psychotherapy profession (current motto: "You're *sure* you were never molested?") and to the nighttime adrenalin-rush crime shows like *CSI*.

Acting independently (while reacting to common cultural imperatives and personal anxieties), these institutions dramatically overstate the amount of sexual violence, sexual danger, sexual immorality, and sexual *freakiness* around us. They've created the illusion of an enormous sexual "other" living in our midst—tens of millions of sexual predators, bisexual sadomasochist anarchists, satanic molesting sex educators, wanton husband-stealing strippers, and malevolent shyster pornographers.

The Industry is continually inventing and warning us about new sex-related disasters in the making. And although government, religion, and civic groups are working overtime creating more and more solutions, everyone agrees that our safety and peace of mind is further away than ever. It would seem that our sex-related problems are just too big, that human sexuality is just too degenerate. That's why programs need more donations, citizens need to be more vigilant, people need to give up more rights, and government has to pass ever-stricter laws.

There's a better explanation.

The contemporary American narrative of sex-as-danger is a rich one. In this well-known tale, our country is filled with pedophiles and date rapists; pornography drives people to destroy their marriages and to commit violence and perversion; sexual entertainment damages communities; sex education seduces children into having sex; premarital sex leads to STDs, pregnancy, depression, and suicide; contraception leads to promiscuity, ruining lives; and abortion leads to breast cancer, sterility, and crippling guilt.

Almost all sexual choices are morally wrong, physically dangerous (for self or others), and economically and politically disastrous. Managing one's own sexuality, or the sexuality of one's neighbors and community, therefore, involves reducing anxiety and minimizing danger, not maximizing intimacy, self-exploration, pleasure, or spirituality. It's a full-time job.

Government hearings periodically bless the latest problem from which we must defend our families. Some of Washington's recent crusades involve "promiscuity," cybersex, and alleged over-reliance on contraception (in the country with the highest rate of unintended pregnancy in the industrialized world). The idea that the U.S. Senate would hold hearings with titles like "The Science Behind Pornography Addiction"[1] and "Open Forum on Decency"[2] sounds like a Jay Leno or Jimmy Fallon gag. If only.

The government selects the witnesses to these hearings who will provide the exact outcome it wants. Junk science, like Judith Reisman's anti-porn delusion about "eroto-toxins," is common.[3]

The basic qualification of many who get to testify is that they're *really* upset. Or a reformed pervert. So ex-porn junkies like Phil Burress create Citizens for Community Values, and demand action about porn addiction. Concerned Women for America lectures senators about contraception causing promiscuity. Donna Rice Hughes washes out as Gary Hart's eye candy and is reborn as an expert on abstinence and Internet porn. It's like credentialing someone as a doctor because she's really worried about illness, or choosing an accountant because he's flunked several audits.

Oh, for some actual expertise: sexologists, sociologists, psychologists. But expertise would contradict the media–religion–civic group–politician Disaster Axis (religion and the media terrify people, "decency" groups offer solutions, politicians fund them). Science, statistics, historical perspective—they might tell us that our kids, our property values, and our bodies are safer than we think. Americans don't want this good news. Given our guilt and shame about sex, problems and anxiety make more sense. So problem-oriented faux expertise ("Look at how I wrecked my life, I know how dangerous sex is") carries the day.

Every industry promotes basic assumptions about the world in which its customers live, and how its products improve lives. Despite a lack of evidence—despite *contradictory* evidence—the SDI has effectively persuaded Americans that the following (unproven) beliefs are principles of modern life (which, of course, justify the very existence of the Industry):

1. Kids are damaged by exposure to sexual words, pictures, and concepts.
2. America is full of sexual predators—and the situation is getting worse.
3. Ultimately, people can't explore sexuality safely.
4. People interested in sexual stimulation, exploration, or unusual stuff, are "them," not "us."
5. Eliminating venues for certain sexual experiences will eliminate certain sexual behavior.
6. Feeling scared about sexuality is responsible citizenship and common sense.

Together, these six assumptions create a landscape of danger and power-lessness, in which suspicion of one's own and others' sexuality is sensible. Surrounded by this much danger and potentially explosive eroticism, fear (and resentment) isn't just plausible, it seems responsible.

This is the context for the SDI's marketing of its products: programs, laws, investigations, new psychological diseases. Allegedly designed to make our lives safer, in reality they make people more frightened. And when people are more frightened, they don't ask questions about whether programs are making them safer—they just want *more* of them. The constant reminders of the Amber Alert system makes parents feel more afraid, not less—while rescuing virtually no kids.[4]

And so regardless of the alleged problem being addressed (porn addiction, stranger abduction, date-rape drugs, blight surrounding strip clubs), the Industry's solutions (its product) always involve the same things: desexualize the environment, reduce the opportunity for sexual expression, increase the costs of sexual activity, increase community anxiety, divide people into the sexually "safe" (us) and "dangerous" (them).

The true product of the SDI isn't safety, but fear. If it were safety, various political, religious, media, and civic institutions comprising the Industry would encourage:

• Condom use among all people, regardless of age or marital status
• Comprehensive school sexuality education

- Regular, ongoing parent-child discussions about sex
- Preventing or relieving childhood guilt about masturbation
- Widespread understanding that most childhood sexual exploitation is done by familiars, not strangers
- Making the new HPV vaccine routine for all preteen girls
- Funding research into the cause and treatment of childhood sexual exploitation
- Including sexual orientation in national anti-discrimination law
- Training marriage counselors, psychologists, clergy, and physicians to understand, rather than demonize, pornography use
- Licensing swing clubs instead of driving them underground

That's just for starters.

The SDI's newest product is fear of same-sex marriage. It's crazy, but of course they predict disaster: straights won't marry anymore, people will demand the right to marry animals or their own children, no one will have kids anymore, children will no longer aspire to couple, too many children will be raised (poorly) by gay parents. As Pat Robertson says, "what about bestiality and child molestation and pedophilia? How can we criminalize these things and at the same time have constitutional amendments allowing same-sex marriage? This is just the beginning in a long downward slide in relation to all the things that we consider to be abhorrent."[5]

It's all nonsense.

If they were honest, they'd say, "We're against same-gender marriage because it's against our religion. We don't think anyone should have the right to do that." But that doesn't inflame people sufficiently. The SDI doesn't want people annoyed, it wants them frightened and angry. It can then channel those feelings into political power and financial gain. Annoyed people don't donate time or money. Angry, frightened people do.

The Religious Right's hypocrisy is astounding. They claim to care about the children, women, men, and families supposedly at risk from the sex-related disasters they describe in fetishistic detail. They tell us to support this or that law, give up these or those rights. But they disappear when it comes to addressing the actual risks Americans really do face—*risks that the Religious Right is creating and exacerbating every day.*

These include the child who's feeling more guilt about sex, the teen who's more vulnerable to unwanted pregnancy, the prostitute who's more subject to customer violence, the swinger who loses custody of her son, the newlywed who can't buy a vibrator, the lesbian unfairly dismissed from her job, and the desperate couple who can't get emergency contraception. They aren't abstractions—theirs are real lives, compromised or ruined by the self-righteous, ultimately worthless flailing about of the SDI.

The SDI's goal isn't to address the real problems of real people. It's to (1) inspire us to fear sex and (2) provide society with excuses to restrict sexual expression. No, they won't fix the problems they say they're so upset about. The only thing they fear more than sex is going out of business.

Chapter Six

BATTLEGROUND: BROADCAST "INDECENCY"

Some people are so upset about what *they* see on TV and hear on the radio that they'll do anything to prevent *you* from seeing or hearing it. Rather than shut the set, change the channel, or use tools like the V-chip or filters, these people are using the most primitive, blunt instrument they can—destroying *everyone's* right to see and hear what they want.

It's a new version of Prohibition, in which a small group of people decides how everyone is going to live. And we all know how well that worked out.

"Morality" groups and too many government officials want something that's unknown in almost any other Western country—to eliminate virtually any depiction of or reference to sexuality on TV and radio, whether programs are free or paid. They present this goal as reasonable, but it represents a radical change in how America is governed. And it represents the triumph of fear over freedom.

The war over broadcast "indecency" is a national power struggle. It's a struggle over how sexuality will be perceived: as a danger to be feared and regulated, or as an inevitable part of life that challenges us to grow, and demands to be understood and celebrated. Even more than that, the war over broadcast "indecency" is about the nature of pluralism: Is *it* something to be feared and regulated, or is *it* a unique and precious part of our American heritage that must be continually protected from both external and internal threats?

This, more than the right to see Janet Jackson's nipple, is the crucial political issue every freedom-loving American should care about. The War on Sex is the battlefield on which the issue of pluralism will be fought. The War on Sex is a Theater of Power.

The very way the public debate is framed—"the problem of indecency"—is itself part of the issue, as it dramatically limits the solutions that can be generated. We could, instead, be debating the "contrast in values problem," or the "some people's discomfort with sex-related programming problem," or the "intolerance problem." Even if we didn't solve such problems, this formulation would be progress—over people frantically trying to solve the wrong "problem," predicting disaster if we don't solve it.

WHAT EXACTLY IS THE ALLEGED HARM?

In what way are the so-called F word (is there a more juvenile expression?), tampon commercials, and talk shows about threesomes harmful to Americans? Here's what the Parents Television Council (PTC) claims, without any serious documentation whatsoever:

> Thousands upon thousands of clinical studies [really?!] show a direct, causal relationship between the messages children see in the media and their behavior and development . . .
>
> Time and time again, we see our children being disrespectful. We hear them using language that would never have been used in our growing up years, ever [yes, the world has changed a bit since 1962]. We see a sexual awareness that at the very least is disturbing [which is not the same thing as "unhealthy"]. What will these youngsters be like when they are adults? Won't they exhibit the same antisocial behavior that is a part of their world today? I'm afraid that is so.[1]

The typical anti-indecency arguments ultimately come down to:

1. Exposure to sexual themes and words is dangerous for kids.
2. Exposure to sexual themes and words damages adult relationships.
3. The broadcast of sexual themes and words forces adults to have conversations with kids that adults don't want to have.
4. Sexual themes and words in the media "coarsen" our culture.
5. "Moral" people deserve to have their "morality" validated, and deserve to have others' "immoral" interests eliminated from the public sphere.
6. Some people are mentally unbalanced, and hearing "bad" words or seeing "bad" body parts might motivate them to commit sex crimes.

And here are the straightforward responses (feel free to use these next time you face this kind of misinformation or prejudice):

1. There's no data to support this idea; in fact, withholding ordinary sexual information and words from kids is bad for them, retarding their normal intellectual and emotional growth.

True, the kind of sexuality typically portrayed and referenced on TV isn't the best for kids to see or hear—it's often stupid, stereotypical, and unrealistic. But that doesn't mean it's dangerous.

2. That's just silly. As a marriage counselor for 31 years, I have observed that most couples suffer from *too little* conversation about sex, not too much. Watching a condom commercial or actors tongue-kissing may make a couple uncomfortable, but it doesn't damage them. If they're so uncomfortable with such things that they have to retreat from each other, the couple's problems go deeper than whatever is on TV or radio.

3. Yes, that's right. And that's *good;* it's called "parenting." TV offers an unending series of teachable moments, of opportunities for adults to talk with kids about sexuality, relationships, decision-making, gender, and values. This is the antidote to whatever is bothering parents about any possible harm from sex on the media. The solution to dumb talk is smart talk, not no talk.

Talking with your kids about references to sexuality on TV and radio isn't a problem, it's a solution. If some adults are uncomfortable with this opportunity, that's no reason to eliminate it for other parents, or to punish non-parents.

4. Our culture has indeed changed in the 70 years since television was invented (and even more so since the invention of radio). During this time, America has also participated in five wars and lived through the invention of the Pill; a huge increase in the number of women in the full-time workforce; a dramatic increase in the age of first marriage; a huge exodus of middle-class people from the core of every big American city; the decriminalization of contraception, abortion, and sex between unmarried people; a huge increase in the daily privacy of school-age children and teenagers; and the geographic dispersion of most families. Oh, and the invention of the Internet and cell phone. If American culture has become coarsened, every one of these changes is responsible along with sexual themes in the media.

5. Actually, "moral" people do *not* deserve to have their morality validated in the public sphere. That's what the private sphere is for. Otherwise, the media would simply be a tool of the current ruling party, as it is in China and Russia.

The U.S. Supreme Court has challenged the very idea that enhancing personal "morality" is a valid government function.[2] Using government power to restrict the content of broadcast media for this reason, therefore, is clearly both inappropriate and illegal in a secular democracy.

6. Public policy generated by the fear of a handful of crazies is *never* sensible and isn't the norm in American life. We don't limit food distribution because of bulimics, we don't limit car distribution because of terrible drivers, and we don't limit the number of bridges because a few people jump off them.

It's hard to believe the sincerity of would-be censors' fear of "the crazies." If their concern were serious, they would have demanded the limitation of private handguns following the 1999 school shootings in Columbine and 2007 massacre at Virginia Tech. They would have eliminated college fraternities because of the periodic injuries or deaths during hazing—but they haven't. Along with "What about the children?" the "What about the crazies?" argument is intellectually indefensible, and we shouldn't give it any weight.

As talk show host Dick Cavett said about TV causing violence and other social problems, "There's so much comedy on television. Does that cause comedy in the streets?"[3]

* * *

One more point about the alleged harm of sexual imagery on radio and television. For decades, Western Europe has been running the experiment America refuses to. European TV features words, themes, and pictures—including nudity—that are prohibited to American audiences and broadcasters.[4]

According to the predictions of America's moral crusaders, Europe should therefore be a cesspool of sexual perversion. But it's just the opposite—their rates of sexual violence are lower than ours, and their rates of teen pregnancy and teen abortion are *dramatically* lower than ours. Table 6.1 shows some convincing facts.[5]

Table 6.1.
Teen Birth and Abortion Rates, by Country

Nation	Teen Birth Rates (per 1,000 women ages 15–19)	Teen Abortion Rates (per 1,000 women ages 15–19)
United States	48.7	27.5
Netherlands	4.5	4.2
Germany	12.5	3.6
France	10.0	10.2

It's what parents are always telling their six-year-olds: "I know you're afraid, but that doesn't mean there's something real to be afraid of."

THEY SEE SEX EVERYWHERE—AND THEY HATE IT

The crusaders who are trying to eliminate sex-related broadcasting have a big problem—they see sex *everywhere*. Where you might laugh (or not) at a simple joke on Comedy Central about penis size, crusaders feel assaulted. Where you might ignore a tampon or douche commercial, they feel assaulted. Where you might be bored (or intrigued) by a Katie Couric episode about teen hookers, they feel assaulted. That's a lot of assault. If you're not obsessed with sex, you might not even put these three experiences together in your mind. You might casually observe "dumb joke + health product + social problem (exaggerated or not)." They perceive "sex + sex + sex." And for them, it never stops; people obsessed with sex that they resent never have a nice day.

When people are obsessed by sex—not about doing it, but by the *subject*—they see it *everywhere*. Like a four-year-old in a candy store or an eight-year-old at a scary movie, *they are simply not emotionally equipped to ignore what they see*. We should feel sympathy for these people, but they make it difficult, because they deal with their upset in such an aggressive way. You know how some people have a frustrating day at work, come home, and kick their dog? People who are obsessed by sex regularly feel assaulted by yet another on-air example of it (remember, they don't know how to ignore it), and in response they kick *you*.

And then they claim it's for your own good. Nice touch. Do they say that to their dog while kicking it, too?

What if such people saw sex everywhere, but *didn't* fear it? It is, after all, possible to see the erotic *potential* around us—sexual issues in health care, the needs of teens to be better prepared for relationships, the beauty of people talking honestly about difficult sexual feelings, the sensuality of babies, the complexity of adultery, the poetry of everyday eros—and rather than feel repulsed and desperate to escape from it, to feel intrigued, compassionate, bemused, and involved in the human parade, the Divine Comedy.

We could argue that moral crusaders *can't* evaluate the "community standard" around sexuality because they don't see *any* sex-related issue *in context* (and seeing things in context is part of the legal requirement for determining the community standard). Consider their outrage about the soldiers' language in *Saving Private Ryan*, or about the shriveled, wretched bare breasts of Holocaust prisoners in *Schindler's List*; crusaders literally can't see these as non-erotic because once a theme or word or picture in any way relates to sexuality, it belongs to the enormous, simplistically monolithic category they call "sexy."

Moral crusaders have also invested magical, demonic powers in certain combinations of syllables. They've spent millions of dollars pursuing NASCAR driver Dale Earnhardt's "S word expletive," Bono's "F word expletive," and Comedy Central roasts that "bring unspeakable vulgarity" into U.S. households.[6] The legislature and courts of our proud democracy have actually spent thousands of working hours debating whether Bono unexpectedly used "fucking" as an adjective or a sexual reference[7]—a legal point that would determine whether the network on which he spontaneously said it would be punished by the government.

Seeing sex everywhere, and hating it, explains censors' desperate grab for power and their desperate demand for action *now*. But asking these people about a "community standard" regarding sexuality is like asking an anorexic to evaluate a movie for its possible connection to food or eating—which they'd see (and recoil from) in every frame.

When the government or crusaders refer to a "community standard," should it be the standard of people who see sex everywhere, or of healthier people who have a less obsessive perspective? We must acknowledge that for people who see sex everywhere, cleansing the environment so that they see none is virtually impossible.

"WHY MUST YOU INCLUDE SEX IN EVERYTHING?"

This is a common complaint of those who want less eroticism in the public sphere. But that's the wrong question, a phony question. And once moral crusaders get everyone looking at the wrong question, it doesn't matter what answers people come up with.

The right question is, "Why must you *delete* eroticism from everything?"

Sexuality is an enormous part of human life. That's why, whether on cave walls, pottery, papyrus, or the Internet, it's been a central theme of art since the beginning of recorded human existence.[8]

The choices faced by the broadcast media (and of all performing, literary, and fine arts) are to portray sexual themes well, portray them poorly, or omit them. Erotophobes want America to move from portraying sexuality poorly to omitting it. We actually need to move in the opposite direction—from portraying it poorly to portraying it well.

Unfortunately, the sexual material on TV and radio is either stupid (e.g., sitcoms, shock jocks) or extreme (e.g., *CSI, Nip/Tuck*). Broadcast media typically portray sexual themes, situations, and feelings as less interesting, less rich, and less sophisticated than they could, not to mention less accurately and more stereotyped. That actually *is* a problem, but anti-sex crusaders don't see it.

We need more everyday, real stuff in between these poles—an idea which, oddly, many observers consider too radical. The intensity of *CSI*-type sexual references may be in bad taste, but it's inevitable. It's how both Hollywood and audiences act out their frustration with the lack of realistic sexuality in broadcasts. It's why the second a show announces that it's pushing the edge on language or nudity—*NYPD Blue, The Sopranos, South Park, The Daily Show*—people rush to tune in. Imagine—characters talking or behaving like real people—incredible!

Methodically stripping sexuality from the public arena not only distorts all portrayals of life, the process itself is socially devastating. We've seen this in Europe's witch hunts, Victorian England's obsession with prostitution, and the "honor killings" of women in strict Muslim societies around the globe.

We must stop being defensive about this and say unequivocally, "Yes, eroticism *belongs* in broadcast media presentations—because it's part of the lives the media portrays, and the lives of its audience." Coming to terms with sexuality is part of growing up. This involves a process that may not always be comfortable, but it is essential for emotional, spiritual, family, and community health. The opposite? Think about turn-of-the-twentieth-century American children who were literally handcuffed to their bedposts each night to prevent them from destroying their health through masturbation.[9] Think about the sexually tormented J. Edgar Hoover and Joseph McCarthy obsessively tormenting the rest of us.

Stories about real life, commercials about real situations, jokes about real misunderstandings—the media doesn't *insert* sex into these, sex *lives* in these. Americans need and deserve to see it and hear it, in recognizable, sophisticated, normal-seeming ways.

Morality groups and many elected Congress members want the airwaves sanitized to be "family friendly" or "safe for children." This assumes that families never observe or discuss sexual themes, and it begs the question of what *is* safe for children; morality crusaders apparently mean it to be reducing all programming and advertising to themes and words that won't challenge kids' alleged innocence.

Broadcaster Bill O'Reilly, for example, believes that five-year-olds can't understand the concept of a uterus, and that the very word "destroys their innocence." He also objects to school children hearing the words "penis" and "vulva" in sex education class.[10] This would give children way more rights than adults—which, by the way, is exactly what these same groups are trying to do regarding the Internet (see Chapter 8).

Decades ago, the Supreme Court ruled that the government can't "reduce the adult population . . . to reading only what is fit for children."[11] Or as Mark Twain put it in his characteristic way, "Censorship is telling a man he can't have a steak just because a baby can't chew it."

The same is true for broadcasting. It's *dangerous* for a democracy to restrict adults to what's (supposedly) safe for kids. It prevents citizens from facing and exploring different ways of addressing adult challenges. It encourages passivity and narrow thinking. But to "decency" crusaders and the politicians who enable them, desexualized adults are less threatening than full adults. Convincing a public that certain syllables or body parts broadcast into our homes are more dangerous than toxic waste across town or overcrowded classrooms down the street creates a constituency that is frightened, angry— and therefore motivated to donate money and time to morality groups and conservative politicians.

INDECENCY VS. OBSCENITY VS. "I HATE IT"

The legal and political issue of "indecency" is confusing for two reasons. First, the very idea of a democratic government giving itself the right to determine what adults can see and hear is bizarre. Second, because this bizarre idea contradicts the guarantees of our Bill of Rights, Congress and the courts have had to erect odd ways of defining what is and isn't permissible.

Speech and broadcasts related to sexuality fall into three legal categories: (1) obscenity, (2) indecency, and (3) non-obscene, non-indecent stuff that some people hate. The three are defined below. If the legal language sounds like subjective nonsense, that's because it is. But our government takes these criteria seriously. Prosecutors and morality groups depend on these definitions to help them limit what you can hear or see.

1. "Obscene" material must meet a three-prong test:
   - An average person, applying contemporary community standards,[12] must find that the material, as a whole, appeals to the prurient interest (i.e., characterized by an inordinate and unhealthy sexual interest or desire);
   - The material must depict or describe, in a patently offensive way, sexual conduct specifically defined by applicable law; and
   - The material, taken as a whole, must lack serious literary, artistic, political, or scientific value.

   Obscene speech is *not* protected by the First Amendment and cannot be broadcast at any time.
2. "Indecent" material, in context, depicts or describes, in terms patently offensive as measured by contemporary community broadcast standards, sexual or excretory organs or activities.

   It is illegal to broadcast anything indecent between 6:00 a.m. and midnight.
3. It is *not* illegal to broadcast non-obscene, non-indecent things that some people hate.

You can see that when a civic group or elected officials want to restrict your access to certain words or pictures, getting the government or the courts to decide that it's indecent or obscene is a phenomenally powerful tool. Once something is ruled indecent or obscene, the government then has the right (actually, the obligation) to restrict or ban it.

The Federal Communications Commission (FCC) could decide, for example, that the word "breast" is indecent, in which case, adults wouldn't be allowed to hear it on the air between 6:00 a.m. and midnight, seven days per week. It could even decide that the word "breast" is obscene, in which case it wouldn't be allowed on any show at any time. Farfetched? Well, groups like Citizens for Community Values are pushing legislation that redefines certain words and images. And already, we take it for granted that Jay Leno can't say the words "clitoris" or "fellatio," much less show examples of either.[13]

As these definitions show, a bureaucrat, judge, or Congress has wide latitude in determining which words and pictures you do not have the freedom to hear, see, or broadcast. "The problem is, the indecency 'standard' is not a standard," argues Cato adjunct scholar Bob Corn-Revere. "It's basically a test for what people find distasteful, which is entirely in the eyes and ears of the beholder."[14] Too much of the War on Sex is described as allowing or restricting broadcasters from doing this or that. While this is accurate, *your* rights to hear and see are equally under attack. This crucial point seems to get lost over and over.

THE FCC: PROTECTING YOU FROM . . . YOURSELF?

The FCC's original mandate was to (1) encourage diversity of programming, (2) make sure there was programming specifically designed for children, and (3) assign unique frequencies to radio and television broadcasters from the usable spectrum that was limited by the technology of the day.

The FCC has pretty much given up on its first two mandates. And now that satellites, coaxial cable, and broadband have expanded our viewing choices almost infinitely, the "public airwaves" are an entirely different kind of resource, which virtually eliminates the third rationale for the FCC as currently constituted.

When the FCC started insisting it could and should police broadcast *content*, it justified its interference because "TV and radio come into the privacy of people's homes."[15] It was a ridiculous argument, but the courts agreed. The rise of satellite radio, cable TV and pay-per-view TV has demolished that audience-as-passive-victim argument.

But under a series of activist commissioners under George Bush, the FCC accelerated its controversial role of government watchdog of what Americans can see and hear. There are only two precedents for this, both disastrous: the 1873 Comstock Act severely punished anyone mailing anything "lewd" (including contraceptive information) and lasted for 100 years. The Motion

Picture Production Code stifled American film production from 1930 to 1968, promising that "No picture shall be produced that will lower the moral standards of those who see it. . . . Correct standards of life . . . shall be presented. Law, natural or human, shall not be ridiculed."[16]

The FCC has blown its original mission—they've overseen the unprecedented concentration of media ownership into just a few corporate hands, leading to the near-destruction of local commercial radio, as well as the news departments of most local TV stations. In 2003, they attempted to pass new regulations allowing an even smaller number of companies to own an even larger percentage of communities' radio, TV, and newspaper outlets. This was such a greedy giveaway that even the Republican-controlled Congress resisted, and the proposal was challenged and ultimately rolled back in 2004.[17]

As public interest attorney Marjorie Heins notes, the public desperately needs the FCC to take its original responsibility seriously—regulating media *structure*, not *content*. It seems "there are a million channels," she says, "but there's hardly a true diversity of ideas out there in the mass media."[18]

So what is the FCC doing instead? Protecting America's children from the F word. Reacting to public "concern" with all the finesse of a 400-pound Romanian weightlifter.

In 2005, Kevin Martin, a lawyer for the 2000 Bush/Cheney campaign and later a White House aide to President Bush, was appointed FCC chair. He says that if obviously "inappropriate" material isn't kept off the air, the very definition of indecency may have to be changed. And he's keeping up with the times, looking at new media as well; he's committed to ending the relatively unregulated state of cable and satellite TV.
Audience rights? Broadcaster rights?

"Certainly broadcasters and cable operators have significant First Amendment rights, but these rights are not without boundaries," Martin said. "They are limited by law. They also should be limited by good taste."[19] *Whose* taste, of course, is the critical question. Our Constitution is cleverly designed to make that question irrelevant by excluding subjectivities like "good taste" or "blasphemy" or "indecency" as criteria for government action. Censoring content according to the vagaries of a bureaucrat's definition of "good taste" is exactly what keeps the Russian media completely toothless.

The FCC has it exactly backward: it favors deregulation of *industry*, but regulation of *content* and *consumers*. They cite the wisdom of the marketplace when justifying corporate giveaways—and ignore it when censoring content that the same market would allow.

Remember that the FCC is required to refer to "community standards" when making judgments of any kind. If taken seriously, this would help prevent the FCC from becoming a bureaucratic kingdom running amok, or from

The FCC Hall of Shame

Here are a few recent incidents involving alleged broadcast indecency that clearly illustrate the seriousness of those pursuing the War on Sex. Speculate, for a moment, on what the next such incident could be. More importantly, speculate on what the impact of that incident would be on America's writers, producers, directors, programmers . . . and citizens.

Censored: New Orleans Mayor Nagin

On September 1, 2005, New Orleans Mayor Ray Nagin was interviewed on WWL-AM radio about the devastation of his city. His anger at the slow federal response and his grief at the resulting destruction were clear.

And they were censored.

Radio and TV stations around the country carried parts of his interview, with his language bleeped:

"I keep hearing that this [help] is coming and that is coming. And my answer to that is BS.

"These goddamned ships that are coming, I don't see them. . . .

"They [President Bush and others] flew down here one time two days after the doggone event was over with TV cameras, AP reporters, all kind of goddamn—pardon my French, everybody in America, but I am pissed . . . "

The destruction of New Orleans last year was a turning point in our nation's economic, cultural, and political history. The mayor's experience of Washington's betrayal, honestly expressed with a few "goddamns" and "BSs," were a newsworthy part of that history—and considered inappropriate by the nation's media.

The interview ends with the mayor and his interviewers in silent tears.

Censored: Garrison Keillor

Yes, that Garrison Keillor, the tapioca-voiced sage of the Midwest, who ends his Prairie Home Companion shows with the wish to "Be well, do good work, and keep in touch."

A Kentucky public radio station refused to air an episode in August 2005 because of two poems containing the word "breast." As in heart, as in soul, as in conscience.

"I don't question the artistic merit, but I have to question the language," WUKY general manager Tom Godell said. "The FCC has been so inconsistent, we don't know where we stand. We could no longer risk a fine."[a]

Was Godell paranoid? Crazy? Illiterate? Station managers like him feel forced to imagine the most prurient kind of mind—and program around it. We're living in very dangerous times.

Chased off Radio: Howard Stern

In early 2004, the FCC fined giant Clear Channel Communications $495,000 for sexual material on Howard Stern's daily radio show. The allegedly offensive material was aired, of course, on a show that everyone—listeners and non-listeners—knows is sexually oriented. Soon after, the nation's largest radio chain dropped the show. "Mr. Stern's show has created a great liability for us and other broadcasters who air it," said John Hogan, president of Clear Channel.[b]

Two months later, Clear Channel agreed to pay a record $1.75 million to settle a series of indecency complaints, including sexual discussions on Stern's show. By year's end, the FCC had proposed more than $15 million in fines against Clear Channel, the nation's largest owner of radio stations.

In October 2004, Howard Stern signed a five-year deal to appear on Sirius Satellite Radio. As a pay-for-listening outlet, it is not currently subject to the same indecency standards as free broadcast radio. If Senators Brownback and Stevens, Congressman Blunt, FCC chairperson Martin, and others have their way, however, that will soon change.

The cost of listening to Howard Stern on satellite radio is now some $200 per year. Until the FCC came after him, it was free. They call this protecting the public.

Preemptively Cancelled: *Saving Private Ryan*

By November 2004, the FCC had filled the broadcast environment with fear. It was increasing its scrutiny of content, assessing higher and higher fines, practically soliciting complaints to justify these fines, and still would not specify exactly what they would pursue and punish. Forced to guess at what would be punished as "indecent" and fearful of the resulting fines, broadcasters became terribly cautious. Dozens of TV stations cancelled the Veterans Day showing of the World War II drama *Saving Private Ryan*—which had been scheduled, ironically, to honor the soldiers who died to preserve the American way of life.

Threatened: All Broadcasters

In 2005, members of Congress introduced the Broadcast Decency Enforcement Act (BDEA). The BDEA is the anti–Janet Jackson–nipple bill that makes broadcasters liable for fines of up to $500,000 for any obscene, indecent, or profane material they disseminate.

The size of these proposed fines suggests a nipple phobia that is simply impossible to comprehend. Can our Congress actually believe the Republic is in such grave danger?

[a]Ken Tucker, "Station Pulls Keillor for 'Offensive Content'," Billboard Radio Monitor, August 12, 2005, http://billboardradiomonitor.com/radiomonitor/news/business/net_syn/article_display.jsp?vnu_content_id=1001014255.

[b]John Hogan, in Clear Channel press release, April 8, 2004, http://www.clearchannel.com/radio/pressrelease.aspx?pressreleaseID=489.

being used as an agent of government tyranny. In continually ignoring this legal mandate, however, the FCC has used its punitive powers to reward the censorship groups that support members of the Congressional Commerce Committee that oversees the FCC, as well as the president himself. By baldly favoring the interests of one group of Americans over another, the FCC has horrifically damaged American democracy and artistic freedom.

THE UNHOLY ALLIANCE OF GOVERNMENT AND PRO-CENSORSHIP GROUPS

People who want to restrict everyone's choices are often active in organizations like the Family Research Council and Concerned Women for America. Others are in positions of government power, like Texas Governor Rick Perry, Kansas Governor Sam Brownback, Virginia Attorney General Ken Cuccinelli, Utah Senator Orrin Hatch, and former FCC Chairpersons Michael Powell and Kevin Martin. The civic groups donate to political campaigns. Once in power, the politicians give grants to the civic groups, or hire their leaders as consultants. Crusaders and government are going after your viewing choices as a team.

That makes sense from their point of view. Crusaders see that their beloved economic marketplace refutes their values—shows and commercials involving sexuality don't go away for lack of viewership, they *thrive*. And crusaders have learned, to their dismay, that their beliefs don't win in the marketplace of ideas either—while they may have convinced many people that their families are in danger from broadcast material, the public still hasn't changed their media habits.

Thus, censorship activists conclude that force—the power of the government they claim they want to shrink—is necessary. They want the government to enforce restrictions that neither the commercial marketplace nor the intellectual marketplace can. It's like schoolyard politics—if you can't bully someone yourself, get your bigger brother or older cousin to do it.

Many in government, unfortunately, agree. They see their role as providing the big stick the anti-indecency lobby needs when its ideas aren't persuasive enough to their fellow citizens. These government officials are happy to lend their power to morality crusaders. Various members of Congress and (typically Republican) state legislatures back this "big government" agenda because they can point to the FCC's work and show their core constituency that they're responding to them. Even the Tea Party movement's leaders are unanimously in favor of that "big government" they claim to hate—when it comes to censoring sexually oriented entertainment, documentaries, and news on TV and radio. Morality crusaders like PTC president Tim Winter then take credit for "cleaning up" the airwaves. It's a win-win for the War on Sex.

In June 2006, Congress passed the Broadcast Decency Enforcement Act, which *astronomically* increased the penalties against broadcasters for "transmissions of obscene, indecent, and profane material."[20] Because there is no objective definition of any of these terms, "the increased fines will create a chilling effect on otherwise protected speech," says attorney Larry Walters. "The censorship will be real, but it will be inconsistent, leaving broadcasters in the dark. This is not good for the First Amendment."[21]

While "decency" and "morality" groups have littered the American landscape on and off for three centuries, there have been few times in our history when they had more influence over ordinary citizens' lives than they do today.[22] Since 1980, we've seen the emergence of Focus on the Family, Concerned Women for America, Moral Majority, and other similar groups.

In 2003, two particularly frightening new players emerged, Morality in Media (MiM) and Parents Television Council (PTC). The FCC adopted these groups with terrifying speed and absolutely no counter-balance whatsoever for viewers who tolerate or want sexy material. According to *Time* magazine, "Almost single-handedly, the PTC has become a national clearinghouse for, and arbiter of, decency."[23]

This cozy arrangement, which recently produced the largest broadcaster fines in American history, was exposed by journalist Jeff Jarvis as government-facilitated tyranny of the minority. Here's the story:

In late 2004, the FCC leveled an incredible $1.2 million fine against the Fox TV network for an episode of *Married by America* that *suggested*—not depicted, just *suggested*—sex. The justification for this enormous fine, said the FCC, was the huge number of complaints it supposedly received.

How many complaints? According to the FCC, 159. Is that staggering enough, that 159 complaints can trigger the largest broadcaster fine in American history, against a show watched by millions?

Wait, it gets worse.

When the FCC's actual data was released in response to Jarvis's Freedom of Information Act request, it showed that the complaints came from only 23 individuals. Reports Jarvis:

> All but two were virtually identical. In other words, one person took the time to write a letter and 20 other people photocopied or emailed it to the FCC. They all came from an automated complaint factory. . . . Only two letters were not the form letter. So in the end, that means that a grand total of three citizens bothered to take the time to sit down and actually write a letter of complaint to the FCC. Millions of people watched the show. Three wrote letters of complaint.[24]

This shocking story is all over the Web—and yet there was virtually no broadcast media coverage. Could the media possibly be feeling intimidated about reporting this, about exposing the shocking bias at the agency that could subsequently fine them and even revoke their licenses? Is this what our free American media have come to?

* * *

Most adult Americans remember the 2004 Super Bowl—or, rather, the nine-sixteenths of a second during which Janet Jackson's breast was exposed[25] during the half-time show—or, rather, the *enormous* fuss about it that went on and on and on. I remember being interviewed by dozens of radio and TV shows, and newspapers and magazines, about the "terrible" event. Parents complained that their kids had been traumatized—or worse, that they'd been forced to actually *talk* with their kids about The Breast.

The FCC responded by both fining CBS and working with religious members of Congress to increase FCC fines for "indecency" in the future. But CBS appealed the judgment as arbitrary and wrong-headed; thus began a seven-and-a-half *year* legal odyssey involving several federal courts, which only ended in November 2011. The FCC lost, and CBS was vindicated (albeit on a technicality). Most people believe the government won't have the stamina to continue the battle; nevertheless, the moment has achieved iconic status. The Parents Television Council, for example, calls it "the Janet Jackson Striptease Indecency Case,"[26] which reflects their adolescent preoccupation with anything that can be considered sexual—and the corresponding outrage they use to psychically distance themselves from their own sinful interests.

In the summer of 2005, the FCC announced the formation of yet another battalion in its war on "indecency." It hired Liberty University graduate

("Training Champions for Christ"[27]) Penny Nance to work in its Office of Strategic Planning and Policy Analysis to "advise on indecency issues."[28] Nance founded the Kids First Coalition, a group that fights abortion, cloning, and indecency in the name of "pro-child, pro-family public policy." Long a vocal anti-pornography crusader, she has frequently testified before Congress. During the 2004 presidential campaign, she appeared on Fox News as a "suburban stay-at-home mom" (a blatant lie) to say that women believe President Bush will "protect our children."[29]

In public talks, Nance describes herself as a "victim of pornography"[30] because she says a man who once tried to rape her watched porn. In January 2005, Nance signed, along with other activists, an open letter to President Bush, complaining of a "huge indecency problem" on basic cable and a growing indecency threat on satellite radio.

The "indecency problem" Nance was hired (with your tax dollars) to resolve is the legal recreation of tens of millions of law-abiding Americans. She will *not* attempt to solicit or provide a balanced view or scientific evaluation of broadcast content and its consequences. She will invite input from sincere censors who *believe*, sincere self-described victims who *hurt*, sincere parents who are *concerned*. She doesn't want input from any of the millions of people who now consume the legal products she will help criminalize. This is not a modern democracy at work.

Penny Nance is now the CEO of Concerned Women for America.

Attorney Paul Cambria has argued many Supreme Court cases, and is past president of the First Amendment Lawyers Association. "What a lot of people don't understand on this indecency thing for broadcast standards is that it's supposed to have a community standard element in it, just like the obscenity law does," he says. "But who is speaking for the community? In all the congressional hearings and everything else they're having, what component demonstrates the pulse of the [mainstream] adult community as to what . . . they think the standard should be? Shouldn't the community have a voice in that? Where's the survey of the community?"[31]

WHEN THE MARKETPLACE TELLS THE UNCOMFORTABLE (AND SEXY) TRUTH

What happens when the morality campaign goes head-to-head with *Desperate Housewives*? In red states, in religious areas, in every single state that passed an anti-gay marriage law, it's all the same: *Grey's Anatomy* is a runaway hit. Ditto *CSI: Miami, Glee, Monday Night Football* and its half-naked cheerleaders, and ditto commercials for Viagra, lingerie, and beer.

Sure, Christian TV and radio sell—but that's not where most people go for entertainment. They're ghettoized, as they haven't succeeded in the mainstream; there isn't enough of an audience to drive "the sex stuff" off the air. So crusaders want to truncate the market mechanism and enforce their taste on the entire public.

They use a circular argument—the marketplace should make decisions except where it makes poor decisions. The media's decisions about sexuality are poor because they're bad for people. How do we know? They contradict "moral" values.

Both our current government and anti-indecency groups claim the heritage of conservative ideology. But "[FCC commissioners] Powell, Martin, and the corporate-friendly GOP have green-lighted big media companies to capture near-total market control over cable and broadcast television," says Ben Scott, policy director at Free Press. "Now, the same bunch is upset over the low-cost, high-ratings schlock that media conglomerates pump into the marketplace. [They] must decide if [they're] free market Republicans or local-values Republicans. When it comes to regulating the media, you can't have it both ways."[32]

As TV started its third decade, 20 years before the Internet, TV critic Clive Barnes put it this way: "Television is the first truly democratic culture—the first culture available to everybody and entirely governed by what the people want. The most terrifying thing is what people do want."[33] Needless to say, "what people do want" still involves sexual themes, as it has since the days of Shakespeare and the ancient Greeks. As proof, look at the PTC Web site's listing of weekly TV shows, which it rates "From a family values perspective."[34] Month after month, those earning a red light are a Who's Who of the most popular shows in America.

How do would-be censors explain this continuing popularity? Do they honestly think people would choose different programs if they had more choice? If so, public radio and TV wouldn't have such a small audience, a fact that free-market Republicans gleefully point out regularly.

Whenever something on TV is punished—for example, the Madonna/ Britney kiss, Janet Jackson's nipple, Cher or Bono saying "fuck"—Americans vote immediately. And they always vote the same—they want to see it. First they vote by downloading or recording the video clip. For example, the clips of each of these moments are among the most downloaded in Internet *history*. And "Janet Jackson is still the most TiVo'd moment we've ever measured," according to a company spokesman, eclipsing—what else?—the Madonna/ Britney kiss.[35] People then vote again by watching the news about the moment and its aftermath. TV stations across America cynically replay the stuff over and over because they know people want to see it. So the moral crusaders' claim that broadcast indecency is being thrust on us is simply inaccurate, just like the claim that porn is thrust on us.

You may recall the fuss over the racy Terrell Owens/Nicollette Sheridan ad promoting *Monday Night Football* in 2004. *New York Times* columnist Frank

Rich noted that the spot was replayed around the Internet and dozens of TV shows for several days, among them *The View*, where Sheridan's bare back had been merrily paraded at the child-friendly hour of 11:00 a.m. As Aaron Brown of CNN wryly observed, "People were so outraged they had to see it 10 times."[36]

The recurring Internet downloading and ubiquitous TV rebroadcasting of taboo moments is *real* democracy in action, not some spam farm that fakes mass indignation. When the FCC fines a broadcaster for violating "community standards," why isn't the fact that the public is actively pursuing the very broadcast moment being fined considered straightforward evidence of the "community standard"? Why isn't it given the same weight as mass-produced e-mails?

TOOLS THEY WON'T USE—WHY?

Media crusaders love to talk about kids—you know, those completely innocent, wholesome, asexual beings who wouldn't even think about sex until their honeymoon if it weren't for our degenerate culture.

Media crusaders want to shield kids from all sex-related content, advertising, language, jokes, and situations.[37] This is a radical enterprise, with a goal so comprehensive that attempting it (much less succeeding) would *have* to create broad collateral damage—which crusaders brush off as a distant, secondary consideration compared with their crucial goal.

What are they trying to accomplish? To raise children who are ignorant about sexuality except in the vaguest sense: That it's an adults-only thing reserved for spiritually oriented, procreating married couples, and that it can kill you or ruin your life. This would make American kids the least sophisticated, least prepared for adulthood in the Western world.

Looking for sex in every corner, searching for "homos" in the same paranoid, bug-eyed way that their cultural predecessors looked for "Commies" a half-century ago, the crusaders have gone after kids' TV programming, both commercial and non-commercial. They've gone after Barney, Buster, and SpongeBob SquarePants for alleged sexual offenses.[38]

The only explanation is that these adults are obsessed with sex. They see it where their kids don't—in many cases *can't,* developmentally—and want to protect their kids from something that doesn't exist. That says a lot about their obsession and their fear.

You'd never know it when talking to decency groups, but parents already have many tools they can use to control what their kids see on TV. Why aren't decency groups talking about these tools ad nauseam? But the goal of morality groups and pro-censorship government isn't really to protect kids, it's ultimately to control what *adults* can see or hear.

That said, here are some tools—most of them *free*—that parents can use to control their kids' viewing:

Off Button

Every TV has one. A perfect solution for all parents who don't want their kids to see something of which they disapprove.

Channel Changer

Every TV has one. It not only takes kids away from what parents don't want them to see, it guides them toward what parents want them to see. And as attorney Cary Wiggins reminds us, "Even though it's called a remote control, please use it on *your* television, not mine."[39]

Ratings System

In the mid 1990s, the broadcasting industry created a voluntary ratings system evaluating violence and sexuality. A monitoring board ensures accurate and consistent ratings. There are seven categories (three more than big-screen movies use) to help parents determine which programs are suitable for their children.

Rating labels appear in the corner of the screen during the first 15 seconds of each program and are digitally encoded into the program itself.

V-Chip

Every TV larger than 13 inches manufactured after 2000 contains this technology, allowing parents to block programs that they don't want their children to watch. Using the remote control, parents can program the V-chip to block shows based on their ratings or other criteria in advance—so the blocking works *even if parents aren't home.*

Cable Filter

All cable TV subscribers can request a "lockbox" from their cable operator, which can be set to prevent the viewing of any channel a parent dislikes. All U.S. cable operators are required to make lockboxes available.

Satellite TV Parental Controls

All satellite providers such as DIRECTV allow parents to easily restrict their kids' unsupervised viewing by blocking shows with certain ratings, locking out entire channels, setting limited viewing times, or blocking specific shows or movies.

"No-Curse" Products

A variety of products can be purchased and installed which delete offensive language from programs. Generally, when a word that's in their dictionary (e.g., "ass," "jesus," "boobs") is detected, the sound is momentarily muted. A substitute word is then either spoken or flashed on the screen. This allows viewers to watch a broader range of programs without fear of hearing something unwanted.

* * *

By giving parents powerful and sophisticated ways to finely tune the exact TV viewing kids can do in their homes, these tools render blunt, society-wide or community-wide restrictions obsolete. A few years ago, the cable and satellite industries launched a campaign to educate parents about these technologies, but this helpful program was opposed by a powerful alliance of family advocacy groups and activists with close ties to major evangelical ministries and pro-censorship advocates in the Bush Administration.

SUMMARY

Pro-censorship groups like Morality in Media, Parents Television Council, and Focus on the Family bemoan the "trash" on TV and radio. Observing the gradual changes in the language and situations being broadcast, they demand to know, "How far will it go? Where will it end?"

The answer is simple: The continuing evolution of radio and TV broadcast of sexual themes and language will "end" when audiences, through their viewing choices, want it to. Despite the political manipulations of pro-censorship government and civic leaders, American viewers are still not prepared to end this evolution.

There's also the trivial issue of the U.S. Constitution that's in the way. God Bless America.

EPILOGUE/ELEGY: FAREWELL TO "TV"

In one sense, this is all looking in the rear-view mirror. In just a few years the idea that TV is important enough to patrol will seem as quaint as the idea of licensing typewriters, carriage-horses, or gas streetlamps. The convergence of your phone, tablet, computer, and streaming audio and video will drastically change both the content of TV and the way that it's watched, the way it has already changed the music industry and newspaper industry.

And so the decency watchdogs have begun to expand their mission. Morality in Media is now obsessed with pornography, sex work, and their alleged connection with trafficking and violence. The Parents Television Council is also focused on video games, cinema, and online video.

There's also an increasing quaintness about the current batch of FCC cases. Viewers horrified by a few seconds of bare butt? Or the word "shit"? How twentieth century. These cases are continuing through our courts because they're addressing unsettled legal principles, not because they're addressing relevant content.

Censors see these cases and issues as symbolically important—an "electronic Maginot Line," as attorney Bob Corn-Revere puts it.[40] And indeed, like the original Maginot Line, all these other media are simply going around the old-fashioned line that the government constructed a long time ago in a different world.

Despite the availability of free, 24-hour-a-day government-regulated network TV, three-quarters of American homes choose to *pay* for some kind of additional TV service (not counting broadband, Netflix, etc.). Somehow censors insist that these people are all passive victims of programming "filth." Referring to the upcoming negotiations over the regulation of cable and satellite service, "It will be war," predicted Rick Schatz, president of the National Coalition for the Protection of Children and Families, a Christian ministry. "There will be tremendous grassroots pressure brought to bear."[41] Tremendous, yes; grassroots, not so much.

These activists who want to comfort themselves by controlling what you and I are allowed to watch still don't get that television viewing is a *choice*, not a *right*.

Chapter Seven

YES, THEY REALLY SAID THAT

The federal courts, and the Supreme Court in particular, have "systematically attacked Christianity."

—*Tony Perkins, president, Family Research Council*[1]

Sex education course materials and instruction relating to sexuality or sexually transmitted diseases should include "emphasis, provided in a factual manner and from a public health perspective, that homosexuality is not a lifestyle acceptable to the general public and that homosexual conduct is a criminal offense."

—*Texas Health and Safety Code 163.002(8)*[2]

America must pursue a civil society "that will democratically embrace its essential moral duties, including . . . caring for children born and unborn."

—*Proclamation of President George W. Bush, declaring January 18*
"Sanctity of Life Day"[3]

"I personally object to vaccinating children against a disease [HPV] that is 100% preventable with proper sexual behavior."

—*Leslee Unruh, director, National Abstinence Clearinghouse*[4]

"If Marriott wants to make another sizable contribution or to build another building in their name, we want people at Brigham Young University to think, 'Maybe we don't want to have a building built with porn dollars.' "

—*Randy Sharp, American Family Association, which demands that Marriott Hotels, which has given the Mormon University $12 million, stop offering in-room adult films*[5]

After taking Garrison Keillor (!) off the air for reciting two classic poems with the word "breast," "I don't question the artistic merit, but I have to question the language. It's not that he's behaving like Howard Stern, but the FCC has been so inconsistent, we don't know where we stand. We could no longer risk a fine."

—*Tom Godell, General Manager, WUKY (National Public Radio)*[6]

"The Parents Television Council does not censor. The First Amendment was instituted to guarantee precisely the type of activities pursued by the PTC: free speech and disseminating information."

—*Parents Television Council, which pressures the government to remove "objectionable" TV shows from the air*[7]

"Hardcore pornography, or material depicting actual sex acts, promotes the idea that human beings can be sexually used and abused without consequences. If we tolerate pornographic material that encourages people to indulge their darkest sexual fantasies, we cannot act surprised when millions do so in real life as well."

—*Daniel Weiss, senior analyst for media and sexuality, Focus on the Family*[8]

"I announce the formation of the Moral Majority Coalition. A primary goal of TMMC is the registration of 10 million new evangelical voters for the 2006 and 2008 general elections."

—*Jerry Falwell*[9]

"We need to yell it to the top of the rooftops that these condoms we're sending down to you don't protect you. . . . [You] have a false sense of security. So I think we're sending the wrong message when we use taxpayer dollars to give condoms out to these kids and we don't tell them, 'By the way, you'll probably be dead at age 24 by cervical cancer. But we're giving you condoms, so go do your thing.' To me, abstinence is the only way."

—*Representative Jo Ann Davis (R-VA), at congressional hearing on cervical cancer and HPV*[10]

"We are trying to create a town [Ave Maria, Florida] with traditional family values and a wholesome environment. That's why we are saying we will not allow adult bookstores, massage parlors or topless bars."
—*Paul Marinelli, CEO of Barron Collier (The town is being developed through a 50–50 partnership with Domino's Pizza founder Thomas Monaghan, who is investing $250 million. Barron Collier and Monaghan will control all commercial real estate.)*[11]

Signing the Unborn Victims of Violence Act, "We widen the circle of compassion and inclusion in our society, and we reaffirm that the United States of America is building a culture of life."
—*President George W. Bush (The legislation gives a fetus rights distinct from a pregnant woman)*[12]

"When two people of the same sex ... adopt children ... I think what you have in many respects is state-sanctioned child abuse."
—*Radio host Janet Parshall, on CNN's* Larry King Live[13]

"No wonder many in America seem to believe that the Court has become one more inclined to protect pornography than to protect religious expression. Most people in America don't believe that God is a dirty word. But the sad fact is that some Americans are left to wonder whether the Supreme Court might have greater regard for it if it was."
—*Senator John Cornyn (R-TX), at the Senate Hearings on Judge Samuel Alito's nomination to the Supreme Court*[14]

Porn users "give lame justifications for their behavior like: 'It's harmless,' or 'Everybody's doing it.' By doing this, they ignore the effect their problem is having on the people around them. This behavior is not OK, it's not even almost OK. This habit is a perverse and ridiculous intrusion into [a] relationship."
—*Dr. Phil McGraw*[15]

"I'm always a little bit irritated when I hear the criticism of abstinence, because abstinence is absolutely 100 percent effective in eradicating a sexually transmitted disease."
—*Former First Lady Laura Bush, apparently unaware that abstinence fails in 88% of teens who pledge it*[16]

"Giving the HPV vaccine to young women could be potentially harmful because they may see it as a license to engage in premarital sex."
—*Bridget Maher, Family Research Council*[17]

"It isn't the American people who are clamoring for more pornography on the Internet and in their communities, and for more sex (including pornography), vulgarity and violence on TV."

—*Letter to President George W. Bush signed by the leadership of Morality in Media, Citizens for Community Values, Union of Orthodox Rabbis, Family Policy Network, American Decency Association, Concerned Women for America, Focus on the Family, Family Research Council, American Family Association, and Parents Television Council*[18]

"Procuring stem cells from an embryo destroys the tiny human being."

—*Tom Strode, Baptist Press News*[19]

"If the public can be convinced that condoms offer certain—or nearly certain—protection from pregnancies and STDs, then the [proponents] can argue that the only thing holding people back from free sexual expression is outdated, irrelevant religious restrictions."

—*Focus on the Family, on why they must discourage trust in condoms*[20]

Those who rent or sell adult materials should be jailed, because, "In the Garden of Eden, the virtue of man was stripped away, and the only way that that virtue can be returned is by Jesus Christ being Lord over our sexual desires."

—*Don Kohls, chairperson, Omaha for Decency*[21]

"The sexualization of our young people is perhaps the greatest threat we face in our nation today."

—*Nicholas Jackson, The Conservative Voice*[22]

"For 25 years, I would have said that the pro-life issue is the most pressing threat to America morally, but pornography has overtaken it. More people's lives are being destroyed on a daily basis by addiction to pornography than through abortion."

—*Rev. Richard Land, leader in the Southern Baptist Convention*[23]

"If my own 16-year-old daughter tells me she's going to be sexually active, I would *not* tell her to use a condom."

—*Denny Pattyn, founder of Silver Ring Thing, popular abstinence pledge program*[24]

Gays "know internally, they struggle with, they know the behavior they're engaging in is disordered . . . they have disordered sexual relationships."

—*Matt Barber, Liberty Counsel Broadcaster*[25]

Behaviors constituting sexual harassment include "humor and jokes about sex in general that make someone feel uncomfortable."

—*Student handbook, University of California, Berkeley*[26]

"Residents should not be subjected to those obscenities . . . They do have a right to have peace and tranquility and not to have this exposure to sex in their face."

—*Flint City (MI) Councilwoman Carolyn Sims, considering an ordinance criminalizing playing porn inside a car*[27]

"The purpose of the First Amendment is to protect the free exercise of the Christian religion."

—*Bryan Fischer, American Family Association broadcaster*[28]

"For many perpetrators there is a progression from viewing adult pornography to viewing child pornography."

—*Morality in Media*[29]

Homosexuality is "the biggest threat our nation has, even more so than terrorism or Islam . . . it will tear down the moral fiber of this nation. And without virtue this nation will not survive."

—*Oklahoma state legislator Sally Kern*[30]

"Sometimes you have to protect the public against themselves. [Sex toys] should be outlawed because they are conducive to promiscuity, they promote loose morals, and they entice improper and potentially deadly behaviors."

—*Rev. Dan Ireland, executive director of the Alabama Citizens Action Program on why the sale of sex toys is criminalized in Alabama*[31]

"The scientific consensus is that every person's life began at fertilization. It is not a subjective opinion, rather a verifiable fact."

—*Patrick Johnston, MD, Director of Personhood Ohio, the group attempting to get fetal "personhood" on a referendum ballot*[32]

"As the toxic waste of obscenity continues to spread and harm everyone it touches, it appears the Obama administration is giving up without a fight."

—*Senator Orrin Hatch (R-UT)*[33]

"Abstinence works." [So how come Texas has the third highest teen pregnancy rate in the U.S.?] "Maybe it's the way it's being taught, or the way it's being applied out there, but the fact of the matter is, it's the best form of—uh—to teach our children." Asked for a statistic about this, "I'm just going to tell you from my own personal life, abstinence works."

—*Texas Governor Rick Perry*[34]

"We're going to have to choose as a nation between the homosexual agenda and freedom, because the two cannot coexist."

—*Bryan Fischer, Director of Issue Analysis, American Family Association*[35]

"I think the dangers of contraception in this country, the sexual liberty idea . . . it's not okay because it's a license to do things in a sexual realm that is counter to how things are supposed to be. [When procreation is removed from sex], we diminish the act. You diminish this very special bond between men and women . . . it becomes deconstructed to the point where it's simply pleasure."

—*Ex-Senator Rick Santorum, seeking the presidential nomination*[36]

"I am not persuaded by the argument that people are more accustomed to hearing these [vulgar] words than they were in the past."

—*Supreme Court Justice Antonin Scalia, in* FCC v. Fox, *blaming TV for "coarsening" public discourse*[37]

"This is just a short note to express my heartfelt thanks to you and the entire staff of Focus on the Family for your help and support during the past few challenging months. I would also greatly appreciate it if you would convey my appreciation to the good people from all parts of the country who wrote to tell me that they were praying for me and for my family during this period. As long as I serve on the Supreme Court I will keep in mind the trust that has been placed in me. I hope that we will have the opportunity to meet personally at some point in the future. In the meantime my entire family and I hope that you and the Focus on the Family staff know how much we appreciate all that you have done."

—*Supreme Court Justice Samuel Alito, to James Dobson after Alito had been confirmed to the Supreme Court*[38]

Chapter Eight

BATTLEGROUND:
ADULT ENTERTAINMENT—
FEVERISH DREAMS,
REAL ESTATE NIGHTMARES

Several years ago, New York's Mayor Michael Bloomberg famously said, "I don't want a porn shop in my neighborhood, and you shouldn't have one in yours."

On the one hand, there's something fundamentally silly about grown-ups running around, tripping all over each other to prevent lap dances and the sale of blowup dolls. The hysteria might lead you to think that dancers, dolls, and customers alike were wielding grenades, threatening to destroy cities in which people don't patronize strip clubs.

On the other hand, there's something profoundly scary about the ferocity of these continual attacks, the absolute self-confidence with which sexually conservative people damn the beliefs and recreation of their fellow citizens. They unashamedly embrace civic coercion—genteel political and financial violence—in a commitment to manipulate government in whatever way necessary to accomplish what they want. Their passionate crusade has an almost erotic sheen to it. If violence can spiritually purify, these people are spiritually pure.

The target is "adult entertainment": strip clubs, massage parlors, art galleries, home sex toy parties, erotic theater, topless bars, adult bookstores, and whatever else is designed to provide sexually oriented entertainment.

With Communism gone, an economic disaster beyond anyone's comprehension, and both immigration and terrorism an enemy no one can fight in his own backyard, lust-and-perversion is the identified menace of our day, an infinitely expandable threat as handy as Satan—and just as omnipresent, if you're of a mind to see it.

Adult entertainment is different than pornography. With pornography, people look at "bad" pictures or read "bad" words, which are *representations* of "evil impulses." The personal *enactment* of those impulses—*actual* swinging, bisexuality, bondage, exhibitionism—is "actual evil."

Adult entertainment falls in between; not simple *representation*, not entirely *enactment*. Entertainment. America has a long love-hate tradition about these transactions: We can't, apparently, live without them, but we refuse to admit it.

Civic censors make a point of calling this eroticism "public," even though it's all behind closed doors and is off-limits to the underage, those who can't pay, and those who don't want it. Not exactly "private" in the traditional sense, they condemn it as non-intimate, stripping it of any respect, dignity, or legal protection. They've been saying for decades that an erotic experience can't be meaningful if it isn't "intimate."

Society desperately needs a third category, a name for sexual behavior that lies between public (orgies in the street) and private (two people behind closed bedroom doors). We could easily call it "commercial," but that's the precise kiss of death in Puritan America. Other linguistic options are "non-public," "erotic entertainment," and "recreational." None is perfect.

As a large group of Americans increasingly accepts and participates in taboo sexuality, the repressive part of society cracks down with increasing fervor. The Internet and the modern lap dance didn't invent this schizophrenic civic morality; it existed during Victorian times, in Thomas Jefferson's home, as part of the Inquisition, in Chaucer's London, in St. Paul's own life, and backward through time beyond that.

But Americans—who typically think "history" is whatever happened before the Dodgers left Brooklyn—see today's conflict as uniquely contemporary. And empowered by a sense of American exceptionalism, sexual conservatives are devoted to winning this conflict by any means necessary short of nuclear weapons.

The ways in which communities across America are successfully limiting their neighbors' expressive and recreational opportunities are endlessly creative, incredibly expensive, and at the very top of many civic agendas. The coalitions driving this are typically religious at the core, but they attract other constituencies as well. These include worried parents, greedy business people, conflict-hungry media, savvy law enforcement departments, and cynical politicians who know a good bandwagon when they see one. Until 1989, the scurrilous political tactic of choice was accusing one's opponent of being soft on Communism. That smear pales beside the power of today's smear of being soft on hard-core sex.

They can deplore the supposed negative impacts on neighborhoods, the supposed exploitation of those poor strippers, the supposed 10-year-olds being lured into massage parlors, and all the marriages supposedly destroyed by husbands preferring lap dances to home cooking. In contrast, everyone jokes about golf widows; no one blinks at the number of blown-out knees young athletes suffer; small towns are begging to be destroyed by Wal-Mart; and marriage, well, marriage is in trouble across America.

So it's not the busted neighborhoods, ruined virginal strippers, kids playing Nintendo with hookers, or bored, philandering husbands that are the real issue. It's sex as entertainment. It's people arranging for sex to serve them, rather than people being enslaved by sexual repression. It's the acknowledgement that erotic novelty is not only desirable, it's possible. And it's the assertion that men and women who choose to use sex in this way can make responsible choices—both in sexual expression and in the rest of their lives.

For those who fear sex, tolerating adult entertainment in their community means collapsing their crucial distinction between good people who repress their sexuality and bad people who don't (and who suffer as a result). If someone can get a lap dance and be a loving father and husband at the same time, the fundamental principle that sexual interest is dangerous is ruined. And there are too many people invested in that principle to let it be spoiled. They will stop at nothing to uphold it. They will use state-sponsored violence, discriminatory zoning, public shame, deceit and misrepresentation, fear, threats of the Lord's wrath—whatever it takes.

Municipalities say this persecution is because of the so-called secondary effects (increased crime, decreased property values, general "blight," increased "immorality"), but it's far more visceral than that—it's having to admit that "that stuff" exists. And some people are willing to destroy the rights of others to make that queasy awareness go away.

What's interesting is that while most people don't feel they have the legal (or moral) right to exclude, say, an unwelcome Scientology center from their neighborhood or town, many do feel they have the right (indeed, the obligation) to exclude adult businesses. There's a cultural agreement that privileges people's discomfort if it's about sexuality. If you're uncomfortable about blacks, you're a racist; uncomfortable about Jews, you're an anti-Semite; uncomfortable about sex, you're a civic leader. Indeed, politicians vie to show who is the most disgusted with non-conforming sexuality, and who works hardest to protect their constituents from having to face their own discomfort about it.

While American courts periodically protect us from those who are willing to eliminate the First Amendment in order to eliminate unauthorized sex, courts at every level have regularly abandoned Americans to the "democracy" of anti-sex mob rule. The strategies that have passed muster in courts include relying on bogus secondary effects; concern for public morals; the desire to limit child porn, exploiting women, and the new favorite, stopping "trafficking." Laws designed to stop "sex trafficking" in West Virginia or Nebraska will have the same effect as the elephant gun I keep in my office: True, I didn't have an elephant problem, but I want to keep it that way. And since the purchase, I haven't seen a single elephant, so the elephant gun must be working.

"We're not a town that tolerates sin," says mayor after assemblyman after minister. But American towns don't actually have the option of *not* "tolerating sin." Supposedly, the reason taxpayers give organized religion so many privileges (regarding taxation, zoning, governance, use of the mails, etc.) is that it provides the social good of seducing people into behaving morally. If a town isn't satisfied with how effectively its churches are doing this, it has no legitimate legislative recourse. In a democracy, people *don't* have the right to live in a morally pure place. They can attempt to live in a pure home, but that's it. Besides, let he whose home is without sin . . .

ZONING

Zoning laws are a physical embodiment of our residential dreams and self-image. But America has decreed limits to the use of this tool. For example, cities can't use it to subtly encourage or support racial discrimination or air pollution. Using zoning to prevent specific businesses from locating anywhere in a town simply because "we don't like your kind" is *illegal.*

That doesn't mean that every community abides by the law. Besides, there are graceful ways to use zoning as a crushing hammer. New York City, for example, has proposed to allow adult entertainment—as long as it's at least 1,000 feet from a residence. In the shoulder-to-shoulder high-density world of Manhattan, that leaves thousands of locations for strip clubs—all beneath the Hudson River. Similarly, ordinances in small towns that ban adult entertainment within 500 or 1,000 feet "of a school, church, park, hospital, residence, or government facility" eliminate every site in town.

If *New York* is considering this, you know that cities across the country are. It must seem almost too good to be true for zealots: "You mean, all we have to do is pass a law saying those nasty businesses can't be here—and they can't be here?!" Other than the customers, business owners, and citizens who value the right to be left alone, who could object?

It's amazing that many Americans complain about government being too big, then feel frustrated when they can't use it in unlimited ways.

HOW A BUST WORKS

Cities and counties across America spent way over $50 million last year harassing adult clubs and bookstores. That's a lot of librarians' salaries, a lot of updated firefighting equipment, a lot of preschool classes for poor kids—*not*.[1] It is estimated that various jurisdictions in Florida alone spent as much as $5 million pursuing strip clubs and other adult entertainment venues in 2010.[2] The *City of Erie v. Pap's A.M.* case cost Pennsylvania taxpayers at least $1 million—back when a million dollars was real money.[3]

Here's how it usually works:

A community has one or more adult businesses—topless bars, adult bookstores, whatever. Each has paid the necessary business tax (often astronomical, compared to similar non-adult businesses), and is generally content to limit their signage and advertising. People who want to find these places find them. Many residents or businesses a few blocks away don't even know they exist.

Somebody decides their very existence is offensive. It may be a politician running for office, a police department wanting a boost, a religious leader looking for a new cause, an exposé by a local newspaper or TV station in search of a story. It is *never* a bunch of people *actually noticing*, "Gee, there's more crime, less virginity, and unhappier wives in the neighborhood of the Kit Kat Klub ever since it opened. Maybe the club is the reason—let's get rid of it!" It's never that way, because that's simply not the reality.

So someone decides to make a fuss, gets some other people riled up, and they pressure the police, mayor, district attorney, or grand jury. Or the police decide to be entrepreneurs, looking for a popular bust that will increase their political and financial support. Either way, several police officers then go undercover. These underpaid, overworked cops sit in a strip club, and carefully, professionally, observe the activity there. They take covert photos. If they're in an adult bookstore, they buy some nudie magazines or overpriced dildos. To get the best quality evidence, they go back night after night, and stay hour after hour. You would too, if you could do that instead of responding to domestic violence calls or carjackings.

When the police voyeurs are sated, they typically close the place down. If it's a shop, they seize the inventory. If it's a club, they arrest anyone they please—dancers, ticket takers, janitors. They note any broken light bulbs or bathrooms missing soap for the scrupulous health inspections that inevitably follow. If only our restaurants were inspected that thoroughly.

Evidence in hand, the prosecution begins. The narrative is always the same: wholesome town versus greedy, disgusting businessman. Sometimes a jury is impaneled to decide whether the dancing or material for sale is "obscene." In other cases, one or more judges rule on whether the business has violated an ordinance that restricts nudity, obscenity, prostitution, or other victimless crime. The city or county will spend at least $250,000 for this first round of harassing the business. If the business wins, the municipality will frequently appeal, throwing good money after bad, often for years.[4]

How much money do municipalities waste trying to eliminate adult entertainment? The *Christies Cabaret* case in Greensboro, North Carolina, lasted five years after challenging the law preventing performers from touching their breasts while dancing. The *Déjà Vu* case in Cincinnati lasted six years. The *Pap's A.M.* case in Erie lasted ten years.

But this isn't a Jimmy Stewart movie with a simple, happy ending. Many clubs and stores win their cases, but are destroyed by the costs of doing so. Pastors who haven't learned to turn the other cheek when it's a buttock say they don't care, as long as the businesses leave town.

Sometimes it works in the opposite direction. Municipalities will attempt to zone adult businesses out of existence, and the businesses take the city or county to court. Local, state, and federal courts are all over the legal map on the rights of adult businesses to exist and the rights of communities to ban them. When businesses spend $100,000 to *begin* pleading a case for their right to exist, they don't know how much they'll ultimately spend, nor whether their simple rights will be upheld.

When courts do affirm the right of adult businesses to exist, locales typically respond by changing the rules: Nude dancers have to wear pasties, or have to stay a prescribed distance from the audience (in a restraining order neither the dancers nor the audience want), or aren't allowed to touch or be touched, or must be clothed when not on stage. One city requires nude dancers to buy permits, which they have to display *while dancing*. They say they're concerned for the dancers' health and safety.[5]

UNICORNS AND SECONDARY EFFECTS: IS ADULT ENTERTAINMENT DANGEROUS?

Concern about the "secondary effects" of adult entertainment is the last refuge of scoundrels.

Americans are guaranteed the broad right to express themselves regardless of the content they wish to convey. Theoretically, the government may not single out particular forms of expression for restriction (like "The president is insane," which is illegal to say in Turkey). Legally defined "obscenity" is one of the few exceptions to this protection. But the citizenry's increasing acceptance of sexual materials in the 1980s made obscenity convictions harder to obtain.

In 1986, the Supreme Court finessed the Constitutional protections of free speech (*Renton v. Playtime Theatres*)[6] by creating a new, *non-content* criterion that municipalities could consider when limiting the operations of adult businesses. This was the "secondary effects" (coined by a dissenting Justice Stevens) that adult businesses supposedly have on the surrounding community. And—unlike in every other regulated industry—municipalities didn't have to prove these effects existed, nor would businesses have the chance to refute these assumptions.

The secondary effects that give local government a "compelling interest" in stopping adult entertainment have typically been crime, reduced property values, "blight," STDs, and a vague "lowered morality."

For years, cities and counties have had the luxury of banning adult entertainment because of these supposed effects. Americans have had no reliable right to enjoy sexually oriented entertainment; across the country, that right has abruptly ended whenever local officials decided it was bad for the community. Some of our most respected jurists were uneasy about this. In 1988, Supreme Court Justice William Brennan warned that the secondary effects doctrine "could set the Court on a road that will lead to the evisceration of First Amendment freedoms."[7]

And that's exactly what happened. For almost three decades, the secondary effects doctrine has been used to restrict commercial and political speech, with cities citing concerns about noise, security, privacy, *appearances* of impropriety, competition, and of course, "harm to children."

Officials in Erie, Pennsylvania, for example, tried for over 10 years to prevent nudity in the Kandyland strip club. The city knew it couldn't simply ban nude dancing, which the Supreme Court has given some free speech protection, so Erie claimed it was addressing the club's alleged secondary effects on its neighborhood—even though it couldn't prove any.

In 2000, a split court used the secondary effects rationale to uphold the criminalization of nudity. Justice Antonin Scalia argued that society's "traditional judgment" that nude dancing is "immoral" was sufficient justification.[8] Justice John Paul Stevens dissented, saying, "To believe that the mandatory addition of pasties and G-strings will have any kind of noticeable impact on secondary effects requires nothing short of the titanic surrender to the implausible."[9]

When experts or businesses challenged municipalities to prove the existence of secondary effects, they couldn't. Fulton County, Georgia, tried. When their studies didn't find the results they expected, the county ignored them and relied instead on old (and ultimately discredited) studies from other states. In 2001, a federal court looked disdainfully on this (*Flanigan's Enterprises, Inc. v. Fulton County, GA*).[10] The county was using deceit to uphold "moral standards." That's what the desperate narcissism of fundamentalism will do.

Unfortunately, the Supreme Court validated the secondary effects concept in 2002. In *City of Los Angeles v. Alameda Books*, the Court ruled, "It is rational for the city to *infer* that reducing the concentration of adult businesses in a neighborhood . . . will reduce crime."[11] The bookstore's attorney, John Weston, challenged the city to produce evidence of secondary effects. Of course, it had none—but the Court decided it didn't need any. As attorneys now understand, claims of secondary effects don't have to meet the same level of factual evidence routinely required in other areas of law. This means that any municipality or civic group that claims such harm will win in almost every circumstance.

Backed by the Supreme Court, municipalities have written their prejudices into law. Ohio's 2005 law restricting adult entertainment, for example, "finds" it necessary in order to protect "health, safety, morals, and welfare," and asserts "convincing documented evidence" that clubs "have a deleterious effect," "lend themselves to ancillary unlawful and unhealthy activities," and that some employees "engage in a higher incidence of certain types of illicit sexual behavior."[12] "Morals," "illicit"—if that's where a law starts, it's easy to predict where it will end. Similarly, a law banning swing clubs in Phoenix, Arizona, "finds" that these clubs are dangerous to the public welfare.

When laws designed to limit and ultimately destroy adult entertainment were examined by the Missouri Supreme Court in 2011, opponents offered statements from law officers, officials, and the neighbors of adult businesses, as well as the findings of academic studies demonstrating that adult businesses have not had the negative side effects cited by the Legislature. Former Republican lawmaker Ed Emery, who handled the legislation, scoffed at the data. He said he thinks it would be hard for anyone who has been near an adult business to deny that it has side effects. "Our intent the entire time has been focused on the secondary effects," Emery said.[13]

In America, laws regulating virtually all industries have to be based on fact. You can't prevent markets from selling ham simply because you *believe* it leads to heart attacks or immorality, you have to prove it first. You can't require drivers to wear seat belts unless you can prove they reduce injury and save lives. But when the subject is sexual entertainment, citizens allow governments to assume it's bad for customers, bad for entertainers, and bad for neighborhoods. That's a fundamental weapon in their War on Sex. It is a ghastly perversion of the law.

America requires police to use science in detective work, and inspectors to use science in making food safe. It's time to require communities to use science to determine if a business actually ruins neighborhoods or harms families. This data is *already* being collected by police departments in every American city; it straightforwardly shows that adult entertainment doesn't usually have these negative effects—which is why cities have never used it, and don't want to.

As far as adult entertainment lowering property values, one club's attorney recently said, "Send all your neighbors to the tax assessor's office every time the tax assessment in the area goes up, and let them say, 'We are right next to an adult business, so our property values must be going down.' And the tax assessor is going to say, 'No, we track this, and the property values are going up.' That would be good evidence for court. There's a bookstore in

Seattle next to a strip club, and the tax assessment last year doubled. If that doesn't refute the idea that adult businesses reduce property values, nothing does."[14] Similarly, when the Phoenix, Arizona, club The Chute sold its building, it had *tripled* in value. Hardly evidence of plummeting property values.

Preventing property values from declining used to be an excuse to keep blacks from moving into white neighborhoods, which our courts have ruled was simply legitimized discrimination. Keeping strip clubs away for the same reason should be similarly banned.

Canada has recently changed its approach to supposed secondary effects. In 2005, its Supreme Court ruled that swing clubs are legal, overturning the traditional test for indecency—whether an activity violates a "social consensus" of community standards. "Criminal indecency or obscenity must rest on *actual harm* or a significant risk of harm to individuals or society," wrote Chief Justice Beverley McLachlin in the majority decision.[15] Some countries attempt to export democracy abroad. Other countries actually practice it.

ISN'T THIS WHOLE THING TRIVIAL?

Is the right to watch a bored 24-year-old gyrate topless really that important? Is a club's right to stay in business where powerful people don't want it really worth the litigation, the personal attacks, the possible jail time?

Yes.

Adult entertainment sits atop a steep and slippery slope.

Powerful people and institutions *say out loud* that regulating adult entertainment is *not* their end goal; they have further plans. Businessman Richard Enrico, whose group Citizens Against Pornography takes credit for eliminating the sale of *Playboy* magazine in all eighteen hundred 7–Eleven stores in 1986, explained this to me clearly: "First we get *Playboy* out of stores, and soon it will be out of people's homes. Then we'll go on to other kinds of filth."[16]

The legal tools they are developing and using against adult entertainment are also being applied against other forms of sexual expression, such as the Internet and "indecency" on television and cell phones. As these groups win victories in adult entertainment cases, they acquire power, prestige, and funding for other battles over sexual rights.

It's crucial to see the connection between the battle over strip clubs and more "serious" issues like abortion, sex education, and Internet censorship. It's the same people, same philosophy, same money, same coalitions—backed by the same political/religious machine. The Family Research Council, Focus on the Family, and Concerned Women for America do not limit themselves to single issues; their goal is a broad transformation of American society.

Is this a conspiracy?

No.

It's worse—it's a war. They are straightforward about their goals and strategy. They *said* they would go after the Internet 15 years ago—and the federal government has tried to censor what you can see there four different times. They *said* 25 years ago they would go after porn—and the federal government eventually empowered a multi-million dollar obscenity task force that, among other things, shut down the largest erotic video arcade network in Texas (over 60 stores, over 1,000 booths). They *said* they would clean up radio and TV, and they chased Howard Stern off of free, *public* radio.

They *said* they'd cleanse every state and city of tittie bars, and they are in the process of doing so. Just look at the following three laws upheld by courts in 2011 alone: In Ohio, there shall be no adult entertainment after midnight; in Texas, people must pay a special tax if they want to go to a strip club that serves alcohol; in Missouri, strippers cannot undress fully, and must remain on a stage at least six feet from customers—who may not drink alcohol at the club. These three states account for 15 percent of the country's population. Other states have their own limitations on consensual adult entertainment.

There is no conspiracy—just a war.

In 2000, Justice Stevens, dissenting in *City of Erie v. Pap's A.M.*, wrote, "Far more important than the question of whether nude dancing is entitled to the protection of the First Amendment, are the dramatic changes in legal doctrine that the Court endorses today. Until now the secondary effects of commercial enterprises featuring indecent entertainment have justified only the regulation of their location. For the first time the Court has now held that such effects may justify the total suppression of protected speech." Further, "The Court's use of the secondary effects rationale to permit a total ban has grave implications for basic free-speech principles."[17]

And there's a meta-slippery slope.

It's not just sexuality the anti-sex forces want to control. *According to them*, it's every aspect of American life. It's all part of a plan, as Dr. Judith Hanna says, to destroy the wall between church and state. For example, the mission statement for Citizens for Community Values (CCV) is "to promote Judeo-Christian moral values, and to reduce destructive behaviors contrary to those values."[18] In addition to a $2 million campaign to close every nude club in Ohio, CCV has proudly created political campaigns to oppose gay marriage, reproductive rights, and effective sex education.

When groups like CCV win battles around adult entertainment, they get stronger for further battles. According to *U.S. News & World Report*, CCV "has become one of the largest local grassroots organizations of its type in the nation."[19] Every victory validates the horrifying idea that morality can be the basis of American law.

Of course, those whose careers are based on policing others' morality are often acting out their own internal conflicts. And so in 2005, after proudly saving Ohio from homosexuality and secularism, Phil Burress got caught looking like just another self-interested political operator. A local group, including Cincinnati's former mayor, filed suit, investigating the clandestine fundraising operations of CCV anti-gay campaign.[20]

And after Burress threatened any Republican assemblymember who didn't support a bill criminalizing nude dancing, 31 clergy from across the state asked the Internal Revenue Service to investigate whether Burress's blatant political maneuvering should disqualify his organization's tax-exempt status.[21]

Fast-forward to 2011 to see a real-life example of this problem on the federal level. The first major hurricane of the late-summer storm season was Hurricane Irene, which caused 56 deaths and $15 billion in damage. Much of Florida was deemed a federal disaster area, which qualified businesses for emergency loans. "We applied to the Small Business Administration for a $2 million loan," says one strip club owner in eastern Florida, "to recover from the damage (two feet of water in the building), put people back to work, etc. We navigated many bureaucratic obstacles, but were ultimately denied based on the fact that the federal government does not give assistance or loans to businesses with 'a prurient sexual nature.' "[22] So much for treating all legal businesses equally under the law. One imagines that the cashiers, waitresses, secretaries, bookkeepers, janitors, security personnel, and sound crew—not to mention dozens of dancers—think that they deserve the same government protections enjoyed by all other American workers. Just like it isn't supposed to matter if a worker's skin is dark, it isn't supposed to matter if Washington doesn't like a worker's job.

In one sense, it doesn't matter in *what* context moral zealots are trying to loosen our rights—we must protect ourselves. If the battleground is sexuality, and some desultory tittie bar on the wrong side of the tracks where more people frown than smile, so be it. Those who find this battleground distasteful, or don't believe it's worth fighting over, aren't looking at the bigger picture. You don't have to have a child in school to oppose the teaching of Intelligent Design. You don't have to watch Howard Stern to oppose chasing him off the air. You stand up for the rights of sad people to watch other sad people gyrate—so *you* can watch, read, download, write, and listen to whatever *you* want. *That's* the American way.

UNDERMINING AMERICA

What is truly disturbing about activists like these is their willingness to attack fundamental American rights to achieve their personal ends: the reduction of their personal anxiety, affirmation of their identity as pious, and accumulation of political power or money. Individual rights that no one would dream of attacking in any other (non-sexual) context are treated as an inconvenience, a simple challenge to the creativity of law enforcement, elected officials, and civic watch-dogs. Communities object to many things, but it is only the patrons and purveyors of adult entertainment whose rights are so systematically limited and violated.

As insane as racial segregation was, at least blacks had their own drinking fountains. But communities are not trying to establish restricted places where people can watch a stripper or buy a whip—they are trying to eliminate such options altogether. And while some observers smirk, wondering who would stand up for something as trivial as a lap dance, no one seems to be commenting on the amount of energy some people are putting into *eliminating* lap dances. In fact, anyone who puts as much time into *preserving* the option of getting a lap dance as people are putting into eliminating it is derided as either an amoral businessperson or an obsessive pervert.

Half a world away from you and me, America is spending mountains of money and buckets of blood to ease its fear about a group of faceless people trying to destroy the American way of life. But from Maine to California, Americans are doing it to America right here. The Taliban would take away the right of a woman to wear short sleeves; Daytona Beach has taken away the right to wear thong bikinis. The Taliban would prevent men and women from watching each other dance; Alabama prevents men from having a beer and watching women dance if they show their nipples.[23]

And the governments of Daytona Beach and Alabama have enacted their bans for the exact same reason that the Taliban enacted theirs: they know what's right and wrong, and have seized the power to make people live accordingly. It's for *everyone's* good, you know.

Chapter Nine

HOW THEY DO IT: AMMUNITION IN THE WAR ON SEX

Those who war on sex have an extraordinary arsenal of weapons at their disposal. It includes:

- Willingness to promote fear, anger, hatred, and anxiety
- Ability to dismiss fact and focus on feelings
- Huge circular flow of cash between government and religious groups
- Lack of media scrutiny combined with extra media access
- Establishment of so-called morality groups as legitimate spokespersons
- Marginalization of moderate religious voices
- Linguistic and category domination
- Explicit policy collusion between government and religion—with many congressional representatives, state legislators, and military leaders straddling both worlds

How could *any* social movement with these advantages fail to accomplish its agenda? Let's look at some of the specific strategies of anti-sex forces. Enhancing our literacy about media, statistics, and oratory may not stop the War on Sex, but it will enable us to see it more clearly, and therefore make it visible to others.

WHAT'S THE PROBLEM?

The very framing of phenomena is the first step toward controlling the conversation about it. Americans hear about "the problem of indecency," "the problem of abortion," and "the problem of pornography" constantly. This means that anyone who isn't concerned about indecency is *for* indecency, doesn't care about children, and so forth. It's far less common to hear about "the problem of censorship" or "the problem of others' discomfort with sexuality," which would make it easier for the public to appreciate the importance of anti-censorship efforts. Similarly, we hear far more about "the problem of gay marriage" than about "the problem of intolerance and discrimination."

Protecting our rights now requires standing up and saying, "We don't have an indecency problem, we have a censorship, intolerance, and hijacking of government problem." As linguist George Lakoff says, "Framing defines the problem. Framing limits what you can talk about. They have achieved the ability to frame public discourse their way."[1]

WHAT'S THE PROBLEM?

Compare these two versions of our sex-related social problems. Note how the definition of a problem determines why we should be upset, and in which direction possible solutions will be found.

• "the gay problem"	Intolerance
• "anti-Christian bias"	Anti-secularism
• "the abortion problem"	Anti-contraception
• "the porn problem"	Censorship
• "the indecency problem"	Repression
• "the adult business problem"	Erotophobia
• "the promiscuity problem"	Moralism
• "the immorality problem"	Religious extremism
• "the sex-is-out-of-control problem"	Irrational public policy

CREATIVE USE OF LEGAL TERMS

The legislators who write our laws can make anything illegal. All they have to do is create a category of what's illegal, and define behaviors that fit into that category. By criminalizing "public sex acts," "mailing indecent substances," obscenity "in public view," material "harmful to minors," "contributing to immorality," and "undermining community morals," various communities have made an enormous range of activities illegal. These now include private swing clubs, lap dances, nude car washes, and, as 21-year-old Clemson

University student Christine Vetter found out, mailing her worn, unwashed panties.[2]

CATEGORY MANIPULATION

Control a society's vocabulary, and you control the society.

Normal conversation depends on many words that lack objective meaning but have emotional resonance—that is, subjective meaning. We agree to use expressions like "intimacy," "frustrated," "overcrowded," "rude," and "in charge," even though we each mean something different by these words. We're all against "sex abuse," but exactly what constitutes it? We all want people to feel "respected," but what do you and I each mean by that?

There are many words associated with sexual problems, and those who war on sex keep expanding what those words mean. "Sex abuse" and "child molestation" used to mean the physical violation of children by adults. Now we hear that adults who go to strip clubs are molesting their kids "spiritually." And we have eight-year-olds busted for "sexually abusing" a classmate by casually peeking under her dress.

A particularly dramatic example of that appeared in Newsweek during 2011. With the provocative title "The John Next Door," the article discussed a single study by anti-prostitution activist Melissa Farley based on interviews with 201 men.[3] Attempting to show the contrasting traits of men who "buy sex" and those who don't, her categories are defined in ways that skew the results—and support her ideological agenda. The "sex buyers" are defined as men who "have bought" sex from a prostitute, escort, massage parlor or sex worker (even once, a jillion years ago), or anyone who has *exchanged "something of value" for a sex act* (which sounds a lot like dating in college). Thus, this category is tremendously broad.

This group is compared with men who are less involved in all aspects of sexual entertainment, have little or no interest in porn, and in some cases presumably masturbate less (she says it was hard to find these guys!). Not surprisingly, she found this second group is less likely to view women sexually, less likely to have many sex partners, are less likely to have sexual conflict with women, and so on. It's the equivalent of finding that people who go to church are more likely to believe in God than people who don't go to church.

But she—and more importantly *Newsweek*—ate it up. They conclude that men who "buy sex" are violent criminals who dehumanize women, view them with anger and contempt, and relish their ability to hurt them. After damning all legal forms of adult sexual entertainment, including the single most common form of adult sexual expression—porn use—the article brings in the artillery: the dreaded "sex trafficking." Yes, an article that starts out bemoaning America's level of prostitution use moves on to the vicious sadistic mentality of the average customer, then climaxes with "sex trafficking." From there it's just a tiny step to "underage sex trafficking."

It's a perfect example of today's Axis of Erotic Evil: the *alleged* nexus that is supposedly destroying America:

> prostitution—
> strip clubs—
> pornography—
> trafficking—
> sexual violence

"Sex offenders" used to describe people who were violently intrusive. Now the criminal category includes harmless exhibitionists, those who solicit prostitutes, and teens who email sexy photos of themselves to their friends. "Date rape" is a terrible thing, but at some colleges, if you change your mind the morning after sex and can prove you'd had a few drinks, you can claim you're a victim. Everyone's language has gotten saltier since the 1970s and 80s, but Morality in Media urges people to petition the Federal Communications Commission about "indecent" words like "butt" and "boob."

And there's the word "child." The War on Sex loves to talk about the horrible stuff "children" are seeing and doing—without mentioning how many of those children are 16, not 6.

Then there are the phony categories used to scare us. It's easy. Take two separate things, one common and one unusual. Put them together and watch how many things fit in. Like, um, "Millions of wives scold or even hit their husbands on the honeymoon," or, "Tens of millions of people leave restaurants feeling too full or even sick." How about these common, misleading and disingenuous categories:

- "Sexual pressure or coercion" (one is subjective and part of dating; the other involves force)
- "Pornography and kiddie porn" (one is legal; the other isn't)
- "Prostitution and trafficking" (one is common and usually voluntary; the other is rare and always coerced)
- "Victims of early sex(!) and molestation" (one is consensual, usually with an age peer; the other is frequently forced, usually with someone much older)
- "Sadomasochism and abuse" (one is consensual; the other isn't)
- "Molestation and unwanted sexual attention" (one is coercive and destructive; the other is a part of life to be negotiated)
- "Missing and exploited children" (one is rare; the other terribly common)

- "Indecent and obscene" (two radically different categories; in most circumstances, the first is legal, while the second may not be)

A popular use of this strategy involves attacking something benign by associating it with something bad: "The F word shouldn't be allowed on late night cable TV because porn is bad for kids." Another popular tactic is setting up and attacking a pointless straw man: "Sex education shouldn't encourage bestiality." Yes, even I can agree with that totally inane statement.

And here's my favorite, repeated endlessly (from Nicholas Jackson in *The Conservative Voice*): "The average age now of exposure to pornography is 5 years of age." I challenge Mr. Jackson to say exactly how he defines "pornography" and "exposure." I haven't seen too many five-year-olds bumping into Voyeurweb.com or ButtBusters 3. If he's talking about kids seeing a half-second of Janet Jackson's nipple, or some of Meryl Streep's cleavage at this year's Oscars, or ads for *Brokeback Mountain*, I can live with this. I don't call that porn, I call it the reasonable life of a five-year-old.[4]

THE LANGUAGE OF WAR

And while we're on the subject of language, here are expressions that are part of the problem. They have an anti-sex message built into them and are used as part of a sex-is-dangerous and we-good-people-are-being-victimized narrative:

Pro-life	Sex addict	Childhood innocence
Porn addict	Cybersex addict	Sex and violence
Abstinence is 100%	Hardcore, smut, filth	Activist judge
Baby killer	Pro-abortion	Traditional values
Promiscuity	Unborn child	Perversion
Culture of life	Pornographer	Normal
Abortionist	Victim of porn	Secondary effects
Partial-birth abortion	Morality group	Obscenity
Pro-family	Decency	Indecent
Homosexual agenda	Christian nation	Harmful to minors

DRAWING CONCLUSIONS FROM ANECDOTES

A week doesn't go by that we don't hear about some guy, present or past, who:

- Has been arrested for rape, with porn in his pocket; or
- Has been arrested for child molestation, with kiddie porn in his pocket; or

- Has been sued for divorce after spending the rent money at a strip club; or
- Pressured his high school girlfriend to have sex the night after his first sex ed class

You get the idea. But no matter how many anecdotes erotophobes pile up, *correlation is not causality*. Just because two things happen near each other doesn't mean that one caused the other. Buying nachos at Taco Bell at 8:00 doesn't make the moon rise at 8:15. *Of course* many rapists consume porn. Fifty million other Americans do, too. Every one of those 50 million drank milk as a kid, like every rapist did. You don't hear people saying, "Milk made him do it."

For a perfect example of this, see Jan LaRue's (Concerned Women for America) piece on victims of pornography, which cites "a lieutenant colonel who admitted killing his wife during an argument about his use of the Internet to view pornography."[5] One bizarre story doesn't constitute an analysis. As heartbreaking as the story might be, it doesn't even constitute *information*. As Alan Leshner, CEO of the American Association for the Advancement of Science reminds us, "The plural of 'anecdote' is *not* 'data'."[6]

DRAWING THE WRONG CONCLUSIONS FROM SURVEY INFORMATION

The abstinence folks report teens tell surveys they want abstinence. Then 90 percent of them have sex before marriage. The decency folks report that viewers want wholesome programming. Then viewers make *Desperate Housewives*, *CSI*, and *Grey's Anatomy* huge hits. Anti-porn groups report that people want obscenity laws enforced. Then 50 million Americans look at porn, and hotel room porn skyrockets when anti-porn groups come to town.

Perhaps these surveys indicate something different than anti-sex groups think they do. They're actually proof that (1) people tell surveys what they think the desirable answer is, and (2) people say one thing and do another. Social psychologists have known the first for over 50 years, and everybody has known the second for about 50,000 years. Of course, when survey statistics are based on heterogeneous categories, the results can mean anything a sponsor claims it does. For example, "Parents favor abstinence until a couple is married *or close to marriage*," (emphasis mine) according to a Heritage Foundation survey.[7] They have the nerve to say that this proves public support for abstinence programs.

Other statistics are abused as well. Lifenews.com decries how both the absolute number and the percentage of American abortions being done by Planned Parenthood keeps rising. What Lifenews.com conveniently omits is that the number of places Americans can get legal abortions has declined every year since 1982, and is at its lowest in three decades. Of *course* Planned Parenthood is doing more abortions. It is quickly becoming the only organization with the money and political courage to cope with the harassment and violence that abortion providers must endure.[8]

WE'RE ALL VICTIMS HERE

Conservative government and the Religious Right love to portray regular Americans as victims of porn and nasty TV assaulting their homes, and strip clubs invading peaceful neighborhoods. Exactly who do they think pays for these products? Or do they think *South Park*, Jenna Jameson, and the local tittie bar are brought to us by altruistic nonprofits? It is staggering that the Right can decry how much bad culture surrounds us, while simultaneously pretending there is no consumer demand for the things they hate.

Similarly, they somehow claim to be fighting an uphill battle against a flood of dangerous eroticism, while claiming that theirs is the voice of the majority that must be heard and given power.

OMITTING DISCUSSION OR PROOF
OF KEY ASSUMPTIONS

The rhetoric in the War on Sex is ripe with assumptions that it never tests or proves—because it can't. It's easy to *say* that kids should be shielded from all sexual imagery because it destroys their alleged innocence and warps their moral vision, but where's the evidence? Without evidence, these assumptions shouldn't be the foundation of endless hand-wringing editorials, one-sided hearings, and apocalyptic states of emergency—and they *certainly* shouldn't be driving public policy.

Here are some other key assumptions of the War on Sex:

- The popularity of porn hurts women.
- "Morality" involves limiting sexual expression and experimentation.
- It's best for kids to be kept innocent about sexuality for as long as possible.
- The value of keeping kids abstinent far outweighs any harm done by how you try to accomplish it.
- Those who want to limit sexual expression and sexual rights speak for the community.
- Undesirable social change is the fault of the various adult industries.
- Porn use leads to violent behavior (although America's rape rate is steadily declining while the availability of porn is steadily increasing).

- Women are not actually interested in lusty sex—such as viewing porn, using sex toys, playing bondage games, or insisting on sex.

Local and federal government hearings feature these assumptions—invariably without giving anyone from the other side a chance to challenge them. Legislators and would-be censors alike describe their opinions in quasi-scientific ways ("we all know . . . " "it's clear that . . . " "the obvious connection between . . . ").

One enormous scam getting virtually no scrutiny is the well-intentioned but poorly conceived Megan's Law. Tens of millions of dollars are spent around the country maintaining complex databases and complicated notification schemes that scare the hell out of people. But there isn't a single study validating that this approach actually makes anyone safer.

QUOTING SELF-DESCRIBED "VICTIMS" AS IF THEY HAVE EXPERTISE

Phil Burress started Citizens for Community Values because, he says, he was a porn addict for 25 years. He isn't alone; many "decency" leaders have led lives of debauchery (a tradition that goes back to St. Augustine). But having been dysfunctional doesn't provide expertise. That would be like selecting an attorney because he kept getting sued, selecting a marriage counselor because she is divorced, choosing an architect because his house came down in a storm, or looking for a doctor whose broken leg refuses to heal.

The real reason these "decency" crusaders are interviewed over and over is that their stories are titillating, and provide the perfect morality tale to reassure anti-sex forces (and it allows the media to showcase its "community concern"). "Look at how sex ruined me" promises a peek under someone's underwear, as well as the "proof" that sex destroys us. Throw in some divine revelation, and you have a moralistic hat trick. If you have a decent bookkeeper, there's faith-based funding in it, too.

The late Senator Daniel Patrick Moynihan used to say that "everyone has a right to their own opinion but nobody has a right to their own facts."[9] Unfortunately, the War on Sex is being conducted by people who are extremely skillful at portraying their opinions as fact, and successfully ridiculing facts that challenge their opinions.

Chapter Ten

BATTLEGROUND: THE INTERNET

The dramatic penetration of the Internet into every aspect of life provides an opportunity to see social history unfold in our own lifetime: What happens when a brand-new technology is introduced into (and takes over) Western culture?

With regard to sexuality and the Internet, the result is frustratingly familiar and predictable. For millions of Americans, the Internet is just the latest blunt instrument with which to terrify themselves and others about sex. And so the most profound communications tool in the history of the human race has been transformed into a battleground in the War on Sex.

Having an existing War on Sex did hasten this destiny (although as described later, history predicts it would have happened anyway). Because the War on Sex had a sophisticated infrastructure already in place, powerful individuals and groups were able to fit the Internet right into their existing SexPanic. They skillfully used the same vocabulary, psychological paradigm, and political machine they had used in prior battles (such as those over broadcast TV and VCRs).

The breathtakingly futuristic innovation didn't impress them. There was nothing modern about the fear they whipped up around it; we might as well have been witnessing the mystery of fire terrifying our pre-caveman ancestors.

TECHNOLOGY IS ALWAYS ADAPTED
FOR SEXUAL PURPOSES

The way the Internet became pervasive in America followed a well-known historical pattern, one that tells us a great deal about human nature and sexuality. This 10,000-year-old pattern demonstrates that new technologies do *not* shove erotic imagery, words, and themes at a naïve public that hasn't invited it, wants to resist it, but simply can't. No, what has consistently happened for 100 centuries is that new technologies are used for sexual purposes *very early in their development.* And that's true regardless of a society's economy, religion, political system, or level of literacy.[1] *These sexual uses ultimately make the technology available to the general public for more general, non-sexual uses.*

One reason for this pattern is that sex is central to so many human endeavors. Humans have an unlimited thirst for sexual expression, health, and comfort. Consider[2]:

- When public baths were introduced in ancient Africa, China, Greece, and Rome, new communication tools, such as pictographs and writing, were immediately adopted for sexual purposes—the names and addresses of sex workers etched into the tile.
- Italian and English emerged as popular, national languages due to the publication of bawdy stories—Boccaccio's *Decameron* (approximately 1351) and Chaucer's *Canterbury Tales* (approximately 1387). Passed from hand to hand and read to a largely illiterate population, they made people want to learn how to read—the languages that had until then been local vernaculars.
- When the printing press appeared in 1452, it was used mostly to print the Bible and scholarly works. But Arentino's *Postures* and Rabelais's *Gargantua and Pantagruel*—filled with engravings of sexual positions, stories of exposed genitalia, and the coarsest scatology—were immediately enormous hits, showing that a press could make money. Although both were banned, Rabelais boasted that "more copies of [Gargantua] have been sold by the printers in two months than there will be of the Bible in nine years." This would apply to every new medium ever after: Sex sells.[3]
- When still photography was invented, it was a complicated, staid affair requiring tremendous discipline from its subjects. But during the Civil War, soldiers demanded their sweethearts mail them erotic photos—a practice so common that by 1865 Congress outlawed it. The new medium of photography then quickly become an accepted part of life.[4]

- VCRs were terribly expensive when first invented. The first videos produced, in 1977, were straightforward pornography; the first non-porn videos followed a year later. People desired the expensive new technology—not to replace a family trip to the neighborhood cinema, but for the chance to watch porn in private. The Sony Corporation predicted videotape would be used mostly to record TV shows, so it created one-hour Betamax tapes. It bet wrong. When the market for videotape proved not to be time-shifting but prerecorded films—porn films—the less-sophisticated but longer VHS format quickly won out and became the industry standard. With porn films available for home viewing, demand for the machines exploded, the price plummeted, and by 2006, 91 percent of American homes had at least one VCR.[5]

Whether a technological innovation involves transportation, communication, or new materials, the pattern looks like this:

- In the early stages of acceptance, a few people predict there will be sexual "abuses" (i.e., uses) of the new technology, which will lead to awful consequences (e.g., cars were predicted to give lovers mobility and privacy, leading to debauchery and white slavery).
- Indeed, people *do* use the new technology for sexual purposes, which can involve entertainment, expression, health, pleasure, and convenience (electricity was quickly used to light downtown cabarets, where people could meet or court unsupervised for the first time; mass printing was quickly used for salacious books and pamphlets).
- The sexual uses lead to the development of practical applications of the technology, enabling more widespread adoption of it (systems to pay for Internet porn were adapted to make Internet shopping possible).
- When the technology is adapted for widespread non-sexual uses acknowledged as valuable, certain groups attempt to limit or eliminate the sexual uses (including inexpensive paperback books, "900" phone lines, and the French minitel).[6]

It doesn't matter which people, which technology, or the format of the sexuality involved, the pattern is almost always the same. People upset about sexual adaptations of technology may blame it on the lasciviousness of a particular group (atheists, immigrants, homosexuals, liberals, perverts); or on the modernity or soullessness of a particular innovation (crocodile dung [for contraception], the printing press, latex rubber); or on the temptations of a particular sexuality (kiddie porn, swinging, sodomy). All are missing the point: Humans are hungry for sexual imagery. They fantasize about sexual opportunity. And they'll do so any way they can.

As people adopt technologies for enhancing nutrition, improving their health, and keeping warm and dry, so too they adopt them for making sex easier, more exciting, more varied, less expensive, more self-expressive, and safer. The Internet is only the latest chapter in this timeless story. And while most humans want privacy around their own sexual expression, most humans are dying to know what their neighbors do.

People will *always* respond this way to technology. You and I will live to see dire predictions, efforts at control, and moral hysteria about other technologies that haven't been invented yet. Because those yet-to-be-invented technologies will be adapted for sexual purposes. Of course.

HOW IT WORKED WITH THE INTERNET

- The Internet, originally developed by the Department of Defense and later by the National Science Foundation, was limited to a small number of specialists—until it was used for sex.
- Once it could actually be used for sexual purposes, money poured into the Internet's development. This propelled entrepreneurs to make the Internet less expensive and easier to access.
- This acquainted more people with the Internet, which spurred demand for access to it.
- When enough laypeople heard about the Internet, some started talking about the "bad" uses of it. They began to describe it with a fear-based vocabulary adapted from other anti-sex campaigns (film, comic books, birth control, etc.): inappropriate content, dangerous for children, predators, exploitation of women, and so on.
- These people demanded that the government do something to limit Americans' access to the Internet, and the Internet's access to Americans.
- To justify this, they developed a full-blown moral panic. They made it clear that the Internet posed a danger so intense that it justified compromising certain basic American rights.

Understanding this historical pattern enables us to look beyond the specifics of the attacks on the Internet, seeing today's battle over the Internet as part of a long series of battles about sex and technology. More or less unregulated until the mid-1990s, when use of the Internet expanded beyond the initial technology-oriented, younger group of early adapters, the demand for legislation to control it predictably grew. *It's not about the Internet—it's about social control of sexuality.*

Consider the Internet's structure. To a degree unknown in the non-virtual ("real") world, the virtual world:

- Empowers users—including minors—and rewards (rather than punishes) them for being innovative and self-motivating
- Presents unlimited, typically anonymous opportunities for sexual talk, research, imagination, and fantasy
- Is an amoral universe, without the restrictions of an external moral code
- Tolerates an unlimited range of beliefs, desires, and imagination

For those who wish to control others' sexuality, thinking, or family structure, the Internet is a nightmare come true.

Not coincidentally, the Internet—in its purest form—also represents the fulfillment of America's loftiest ideals:

- Democracy: equal rights for all participants
- Meritocracy: no one cares about your "actual" skin color or "true" physical beauty
- Liberal rights: people can do whatever they want if they're not hurting others
- Pluralism: the recognition that different people want different things, and the assumption that all will tolerate all

These are two different ways of describing the same phenomenon. Many people hate or fear the Internet precisely because it fulfills these lofty American ideals.

HISTORY OF THE INTERNET

The Internet started out as part of a multi-nation physics research project, CERN. Computers had been around since the end of World War II. By the 1950s, deep in the Cold War, the U.S. government wondered how to keep its chain of command intact in the event of a nuclear war. The desired solution was to have a decentralized system that didn't physically exist anywhere. That system became the Internet. It won't, of course, survive a nuclear war, and today's typical Internet user rarely thinks about its military uses.

At first, participating in the Internet required technical skill and equipment that few people had or could acquire. The early participants were an esoteric group, members of a mostly invisible subculture that developed its own language, etiquette, and priorities.

During the 1980s, a long series of technical achievements was making the Internet more practical for more people. Things we take for granted today had to be, and were, invented: HTML, URLs. The World Wide Web project was announced in 1991. Three years later, Netscape released the first browser.

And the thing that drove the whole development was . . . sex. Pornography to look at. To read. To buy. Chat rooms in which to discuss sex or have "virtual" sexual experiences. Fetish sites that proved you weren't the only one who enjoyed your unusual fantasy. E-mail with which people could flirt, discuss sex, and masturbate together. People took pictures of themselves nude or having sex and posted them for others to enjoy (today when teens do that, it's called sexting). Online pornography was the first consistently successful e-commerce product.

With the Internet becoming more easily usable, people started going to it for a wide range of non-sexual activities: shopping (made possible because of porn-for-pay systems), research (via the high-resolution, compressed images needed for porn), education (via the CD-ROMs developed to deliver porn), and e-mail for worldwide communication (a network financed by people using it for sexual purposes).

And so the whole country started finding out about this cool way to interact with others. And some people started freaking out about the way it could be used to interact sexually with others. Which brings us to the predictable thing that happened next: People brought the War on Sex to the Internet. The frontline moved online.

THE MORAL PANIC OVER THE INTERNET

It wasn't long before the public was being told there was "too much" sex on the Internet, and that it posed a danger to many people, particularly children. There was already a powerful civic-political alliance battling against sexual rights relating to videotape, TV, radio, telephone sex, library books, and adult entertainment. Thus, there was an infrastructure of fear/danger already in place to claim that:

- Sexual material on the Internet is dangerous.
- An ever-growing group of people were "abusing" the new technology, increasing kids' vulnerability.
- These people were themselves dangerous.

The supposedly out-of-control reader of nasty comics and graphic novels was simply transformed into the out-of-control reader of Internet porn. The supposedly ever-present playground predator was easily transformed into the ever-present chat-room predator.

Since the special technology of the Internet makes an enormous range of words and images widely available, people who worried about uncontrolled access and experience were easily frightened. Sexual imagery formed an easy target on which to focus the anxiety of this group; for anyone who believes that access to the "wrong" material frees people's dangerous "latent tendencies," the Internet is the most treacherous thing ever invented.

Many institutions—churches, "morality" groups, think tanks, parent groups—devoted themselves to controlling online sexuality, while many more came into being with this specific mission. It was the focus of enormously successful fundraising efforts; indeed, it helped make some groups, like Concerned Women for America and Focus on the Family, the big players they are today. Like Jenna Jameson and then-Senator, now Governor Sam Brownback, they can proudly say they owe their success to Internet porn.

Since the constituents of these crusading groups were (and often still are) technologically unsophisticated, they were easily misled about the magnitude of the dangers the Internet posed. Those already participating in other moral panics (regarding, for example, homosexuality, child abduction, satanic abuse, feminism, or contraception) found it easy to believe almost any assertion about destructive sex on the Web.

If they heard sensational claims about it, they rarely checked them out and certainly weren't having experiences that contradicted these lies. If their pastor told them that kids can access millions of Web sites showing women having sex with horses, they didn't surf the Web to discover it isn't true. If they heard that there are perverts molesting young girls in every chat room in cyberspace, they didn't go to chat rooms with their nieces and share benign experiences there.

The moral panic was fed by stories citing the explosive availability of, and interest in, sexual material on the Internet. It became commonplace to cite how sex was the most-searched-for word on the Internet, a fact that has continued to this day. Of course.

Naturally, tens of millions of people, from every walk of American life, were eager to look at, think about, or discuss sex via the Internet. But anti-sex forces didn't consider the meaning of this very typical interest. Instead, the moral panic quickly grew to the point where some people demanded that the government take steps to control what *others* could see, read, and hear on the Internet. Congress responded with a series of measures in 1995 and 1996, claiming to protect children from "computer pornography," material "harmful to minors," and the use of morphing technology to create simulated child porn.

The Communications Decency Act of 1996 was struck down the following year for being unconstitutionally vague. But people were still fearful (or were pandering to those who were), and yearned for more control over the Internet.

In 1998, Senator John McCain (R-AZ) introduced legislation "to ensure that pervasive, obscene, and violent material is screened out [of schools and libraries] and that our children are protected."[7] The government ultimately passed the outlandishly comprehensive Child Online Protection Act (COPA), which criminalized the sending of anything "harmful to minors" (which has no precise legal meaning, and is generally protected by the First Amendment) over the Internet.

So the government joined in the Big Lie about (1) the Internet being a dangerous environment that (2) needed to be controlled. That Big Lie is now about predators and "trafficking." Same nonsense.

The moral panic around the Internet needed villains, of course. Not surprisingly, the category of "dangerous people" has grown bigger and bigger. It now includes couples who post nude photos of themselves; college students who complain bitterly about school, teachers, or each other; adult women who dress in fantasy teenager costumes; impolite bloggers; and people who publish information about sexual health, homosexuality, and non-monogamy.

Anti-sex forces continually expressed outrage that so-called pornographers were allowed to do what they wanted on the Internet—as if the rights of people to consume what pornographers were producing was of no importance. So pornographers were a handy villain. And the people who protected Americans' rights to consume their online products—such as the American Civil Liberties Union, National Coalition Against Censorship, and People for the American Way—were branded as protecting pornographers' rights to poison America.

That strategy has continued to this very day—ignoring the rights of consumers of sexually oriented materials when discussing possible harm and possible solutions.

A SPECIAL KIND OF PANIC—STATE BY STATE

As the panic spread, the Internet was increasingly looked upon as an enormous pipeline pumping toxic sewage into innocent homes, giving psychotic predators access to innocent lives. This fantasy persists in the way porn is described by anti-porn activists today—that it's being pumped into homes where it isn't wanted.

Individual states began passing laws attempting to prevent this monstrous technology from harming its citizens.Pennsylvania's law is typical. Passed in 2002, it required all Internet service providers (ISPs) to block access to sites *accused* of containing child pornography. The state attorney general, or any county district attorney, could ask a local judge to declare that a certain Web site *might* be child pornography, thus requiring any ISP serving Pennsylvania citizens to block it. This would occur with no prior notice to the ISP or Web site owner, with no option of appeal.

The law imposed potential liability on ISPs, even if they had no relationship with the publishers of the allegedly offensive content. *Any ISP doing business in Pennsylvania was therefore potentially liable for content anywhere on the Internet.*

Not satisfied, Pennsylvania's attorney general started issuing orders directly to ISPs—over 300—demanding they block certain content. But he refused to disclose the content of these secret orders. So for a year, providing Internet service in Pennsylvania was a dangerous business. Residents never knew which sites they couldn't access due to mere suspicion, or worse, because an innocent Web site was technically entangled with a site that was suspected. Finally, the law was overturned in court in 2004. Nevertheless, other states (including Arizona, New York, and Michigan) eventually passed similar laws, all of which were struck down. A new Massachusetts law was challenged in 2010, and was only settled in 2011.

Pennsylvania's law was technologically impossible and constitutionally unacceptable. But it did make a statement: We are so afraid of child porn that we're willing to shut down the Internet in Pennsylvania.[8]

FILTERING? BLOCKING? CENSORING? YOUR EYES ARE THE BATTLEFIELD

Just as fear of alcohol (particularly of how immigrants, poor people, and minors were using it) 80 years ago led to Prohibition, fear of the Internet (particularly of how perverts, liberals, and minors were using it) led to demands for "filtering" technology.

This was the impetus for developing Internet filtering software, which many private companies made commercially available starting in the mid-1990s. Installed on a computer, it would prevent the user from accessing Web sites whose address or content were considered "inappropriate"—that is, connected with sexuality. Vendors claimed that their products "protected children" by eliminating "pornographic" content, but the range of sexual references they eliminated was extraordinarily wide. This included sites about breast cancer, psychology, political debate, art, and even people (Dick Armey) and communities (Middlesex) whose names included certain magic letters.[9] MapleSoccer.org was blacklisted by CyberPatrol because it listed teams as "boys under 12," "boys under 10," and so on. And in the ultimate irony, FilteringFacts.org (a pro-censorship site) was blocked by SurfWatch, one of the most popular blocking programs in the country.

These companies did what any profit-making venture does: they encouraged a demand for their product. Logically, they did so by "alerting" people to the terrible dangers cyberspace posed—mostly for their children, but even for themselves. Note, for example, the description on this site selling a variety of filtering products:

> Today's high-tech porn pushers are more aggressive than ever before, making it almost impossible to protect our families from unwanted pornography. Thankfully, with tools like Internet filtering software, it's possible to fight back.[10]

Note the language: "porn-pushers" are "aggressive," we need to "protect our families," and now we can "fight back." This site sells fear, need, and a solution in just two sentences.

Thus, these companies were in collusion with people and groups whose agenda is to frighten the public about the sexual uses of the Internet. That has continued to this day, primarily because they have a common goal—to raise alarm about the sexual aspects of the Internet—and also because the institutions of the Right purchase and encourage the use of these products. For example, religious and other conservative groups increasingly urge the use of filtering software as part of the treatment of "porn addiction" and "cybersex addiction." CYBERsitter was once distributed by the anti-porn group Focus on the Family. The site FilteringFacts.org, purporting to explain the facts supporting filtering, was partly funded by the group Enough Is Enough, whose stated mission is protecting children and families from Internet porn.[11]

In selling security products such as burglar alarms and motion detectors, the key to success is persuading potential customers that they are vulnerable. People, of course, are more easily frightened by appeals to emotion than by fact. And so filtering companies, like their anti-sex collaborators, recklessly repeat new wives' tales, such as "The average age a child is first exposed to pornography online is 11 years old," and, "Nearly all (90 percent) kids aged 8 to 16 have viewed porn online, mostly while doing homework."[12]

These numbers are created via categories so broad that they show almost everyone experiencing almost everything. For example, according to ProtectYourKids.info, "More than half of teenagers have visited Internet sites containing pornography, offensive music lyrics, gambling or messages of violence or hate." Only half? With a category that diverse, 99 percent is probably more like it. Looking at scary data just a bit clarifies it a great deal. A 2000 "online victimization" study by the National Center for Missing and Exploited Children (www.ncmec.org) reveals that 96 percent of those who solicit teens are under 25, and nearly half are themselves children under the age of 18.

Having succeeded in persuading the public that their product is desperately needed, filtering companies sold it, while refusing to tell people exactly what they were buying. What were their algorithms? What words, sites, concepts were blocked? How did they add or delete a site? Every filtering company had the same response: That's proprietary information, and we're not telling.

There's nothing wrong with the manufacturer of Coca-Cola saying that, because no one is forced to buy their product, and Coke isn't needed in order to do your job, get proper health care, acquire an education, or be an effective citizen. But when your employer, library, hospital, city planner, or university is *required* to use a filtering company's product as part of using their computer, or consumers of these institutions are subject to the limitations of filtering products (a doctor can't find out about the health issues involved in anal sex, a library can't provide information about the longevity of non-monogamous couples, a city planner can't find out about zoning and prostitution, a judge isn't allowed to read about sadomasochism being discussed in a case),[13] "we won't discuss our product" is outrageous and inappropriate.

Private companies enjoying the huge advantages of being used as quasi-public utilities should be required to disclose substantial product information. But presumably, any government that required this transparency wouldn't be requiring Internet filtering in the first place.

Was there really a problem? Morality groups cried yes, although no one could really point to much actual harm. In congressional testimony on November 10, 1998, they told satanic stories of an 11-year-old boy "hooked on pornography" who "left semen samples in his favorite teacher's cup," and a babysitter showing porn to a four-year-old who then wrote "sexually explicit notes to a little girl in his first grade class."[14] And unfortunately, their fear drove public policy decisions in Congress. How is it that being frightened is its own credential to discuss sexuality and behavioral science?

Filtering was a solution looking for a problem, according to the federal District Court that overruled the Loudon County (Virginia) library's use of filtering that very year (1998):

> No reasonable trier of fact could conclude that three isolated incidents nationally, one very minor isolated incident in Virginia, no evidence whatsoever of problems in Loudon County, and not a single employee complaint from anywhere in the country establish that the [filtering] policy is necessary to prevent sexual harassment or access to obscenity or child pornography.[15]

Nevertheless, by 1997 the group Family Friendly Libraries identified its top priority as "protecting children from age-inappropriate materials." Chaired by Phil Burress—who went on to promote laws prohibiting same-gender marriage, adult entertainment establishments, and any advertising that "exploits" sexuality—they demanded the installation of filtering systems in public libraries.[16] And did the corporate rationale of "proprietary information" justify the compromise of library patrons' rights? Not according to the federal court that overturned the Loudon County library's filtering policy: "A defendant cannot avoid its constitutional obligation by contracting out its decision-making to a private entity."[17]

The collusion between filtering companies, the Right, and the government reached its zenith in 2000 with the Child Internet Protection Act (CIPA), passed after federal courts overturned two congressional attempts to censor the Internet.[18] CIPA required libraries to install Internet filtering—even for adults—if they wanted to receive federal funds. Undereducated in the meaning of American democracy, ignoring the critical mandate of public schools to encourage curiosity, most city councils and county supervisors thought the funding was more important than whatever material would be excluded. Besides, no elected official wanted to be in the position of sacrificing desperately needed funds so that patrons could "look at porn all day long."

Some libraries didn't even wait for the federal demand to install filters. The Kern County, California, library had to be threatened with legal action in January 1998 if they didn't remove the filtering software. Less than a year later, a federal judge ruled that a library in Loudon County, Virginia, had to reverse its policy of installing filters on its computers.[19]

CIPA exposed any pretense of so-called conservatives of simply wanting to raise their families and live their lives free from government intrusion. Any parent concerned about library computers can take their kids to the library and supervise them, or forbid their kids from going to a library alone. Instead, these "conservatives" brought a system to every town in America in which the government—implementing their personal values—controlled what everyone could see and hear.

They had done it before with adult bookstores, strip clubs, and video shops. But this was the most naked attack on democracy yet—bringing censorship to public libraries. You might as well melt down the Statue of Liberty and use the metal to fashion jail bars, or chastity belts for the mind. To these people, Americans don't deserve their basic rights if they use them in the context of sexuality.

But exactly what criteria these blocking systems would use, or what they would block, no one knew—no librarian, no senator, no parent. All anyone knew is that these filtering systems promised to protect children *and* adults from material unsuitable for minors. In reality, *there was no category of non-objectionable sexual references*. No health, educational, legal, political, historical, or even religious reference to sexuality could get through the electronic censor. Filtering products attempt to create an Internet in which sexuality doesn't exist, as if there's no such thing as a legitimate or non-dangerous interest in sexuality. That was, and still is, an explicit goal of the War on Sex.

Even the court *upholding* CIPA recognized that "a filter set to block pornography may sometimes block other sites that present neither obscene nor pornographic material"—in other words, *legal* material.[20] The Court just didn't think that adults losing access to legal material (called "censorship" when done in countries we don't like) was as important as "protecting" young people from certain words or pictures.

In dissenting, Justice Stevens took the loss of access to legal material seriously   properly ignoring the fact that much of it was about sexuality: "The Children's Internet Protection Act (CIPA) operates as a blunt nationwide restraint on adult access to an enormous amount of valuable information that individual librarians cannot possibly review . . . *Most of that information is constitutionally protected speech.* In my view, this restraint is unconstitutional."[21]

So what do filters filter out? As filtering became more popular, thousands of examples of what filtering actually did quickly accumulated. Here's a sample of what some popular programs blocked access to:

- CyberPatrol blocked the book *Sex, Laws and Cyberspace.*
- CYBERsitter blocked the National Organization for Women's Web site.
- SurfControl blocked the "emotional changes" section of Kotex.com.[22]
- Websense blocked the Web site of A Different Light Bookstore.
- N2H2 blocked the Web site of the Rape Crisis Center of Central Massachusetts.[23]
- Tens of thousands of Web sites with *no* sexual content whatsoever were blocked if their URLs happen to share a numerical Internet protocol address with a pornography site.
- During the 2000 election, numerous candidates' Web sites were blocked, including Jeffrey Pollack's. Running for Congress in Oregon, his site said, "We should demand that all public schools and libraries install and configure Internet Filters"—until he discovered *he* was filtered, and changed his position.[24]

These are programs being used in public libraries across the United States. They are ammunition in the War on Sex.[25]

According to their study, says Will Doherty, Executive Director of the Online Policy Group, "For every web page blocked as advertised, there was collateral damage of at least one other page improperly blocked."[26]

It is important to understand that this "collateral damage" is *not* an anomaly—it is the way filtering software works. The question is, is this acceptable? Exactly how much is America willing to pay to protect young eyes from something whose damage hasn't really been studied, and has certainly never been proven? What this tool unintentionally deletes isn't porn or danger or sex, it's information, and it's the freedom to acquire information. This is what the War on Sex is about.

This would be bad enough if that were the extent of it. But it isn't. For starters, you can't know something is filtered out if you don't look for it. You may not realize there's another side to a medical or political story. In 2011, for example, there were major news stories questioning the necessity for the current prostate cancer screening test; two years before that, the value of routine mammograms was questioned. Next year, as this year, the legal penalties for teen sexting will be debated in various state legislatures. None of these news stories would make it through certain Internet blocking software—and the user wouldn't know they'd been censored.

And there are a lot of sites that get filtered out for purely political reasons: sites of gay sports clubs, for example, which don't discuss homosexuality; sites involving nuclear disarmament. When filtering company CyberPatrol was confronted with why right-wing hate sites weren't listed as such, they had no good answer. When Peacefire publicized this, CyberPatrol went after *them*. In fact, when Peacefire started posting essays on its Web site critical of filtering software, some software companies such as CYBERsitter reacted by blocking Peacefire's Web site—which contained neither pornography nor sexual words. And when *Time* magazine criticized CYBERsitter for blocking its critics' sites, CYBER-sitter blocked *Time*'s site. There will always be a political agenda with blocking software.[27] If these private companies are living off the quasi-public teat, this is unacceptable.

Perhaps worst of all is when computer users use filters unwillingly, or even unknowingly. One common way this happens is when blocking software is placed on the computer you use by the person or institution that controls it. This can be your employer, city council, hospital, school, or whomever sets policy where you use it. Sites may not come up when you search a topic, or, more generally, they come up but you can't access them. Similarly, if you type in a URL that's blocked by a decision beyond your control, you get an error message, or are told the site is unavailable, when it actually is available—just not to you. This is exactly how Internet cafes operate in China today.

In late 2005, while my own computer was being repaired, I discovered that both my Web sites (www.SexualIntelligence.org, www.SexEd.org) were blocked on the computers that customers rent at FedEx Kinko's—all 1,200 locations. How many tens of thousands of people across the United States (and the world) had searched for words or ideas they could have found on one of my sites—if they hadn't been blocked?

When I inquired about this, I was directed to the company Kinko's had hired to do the blocking. They were very nice, and offered to review my sites. They eventually said my sites had been blocked by "an oversight"—the same thing all producers of non-porn sites are told when they discover their work has been blocked. The vaunted technical capacity and "human review" of filtering products simply cannot do what the companies promise. And since their financial incentive is to overblock rather than underblock, this fundamental inadequacy will not change.

You're probably also a consumer of blocking software through your ISP. AOL, Yahoo!, and most others have "user guidelines" or "user agreements" (you did read the miles of fine print, right?) that basically say they'll filter out anything they don't like, and that they're not obligated to tell you what, why, or when. And so AOL has booted the *Triangle News* gay newspaper site. Yahoo! closed a variety of sexuality and gender support groups, such as SF Queer Longhairs.[28]

Similarly, Microsoft's blogging tool MSN Spaces censors certain words you might try to include in a blog title or URL. In Xeni Jardin's 2004 experiment, blog titles refused include "Corporate Whore," "Pornography & the Law," and most anything with the traditional "seven dirty words" the Federal Communications Commission won't let you say on network TV.[29] On the other hand, the software allowed "World of Poop" and "Butt Sex is Awesome." It didn't allow "Anal Health for People who Think Buttsex is Awesome," however. All of which shows that filtering software doesn't make kids safer, it just gives them more reasons to disrespect efforts to censor what they read. Which is, ultimately, the effect of all censorship. And as America learned during the drug wars of the 1960s, any government policy whose main effect is creating disrespect for the government is a bad policy.

But here's something cheery—circumvention technology, distributed by groups like Peacefire.org and activists like Bennett Haselton. These are programs used by people to get around the blocking software that's been installed in their schools or workplaces, and by users in countries where the Internet is censored. "In a nice twist," reports technology access expert Haselton, "the ad revenue that comes from users in countries like the U.S. helps to fund the services that provide circumvention to people in countries like Iran and China."

THE GOVERNMENT'S ATTEMPTS TO CONTROL YOUR ACCESS TO THE NET

From the moment the Internet became a popular medium, local and federal government attempted to limit Americans' access to it—and they've kept at it to this very day. The three most popular charges have been "child pornography" (the definition of which keeps expanding), "obscenity" (a subjective category that can only be defined by a jury that determines the "community standards" allegedly violated), and "harmful to minors" (an arbitrary category that has never actually been defined).

Pressured by conservative, religious, and feminist groups, the government has continuously assumed there is harm posed by the Internet, and has consistently attempted to limit this alleged harm by limiting both adults' and minors' access to it. Not only has the alleged harm never been proven, the effectiveness of censoring the Internet in limiting this alleged harm has never been demonstrated. Instead, the "common sense" of one part of the community has substituted for the science they don't have and the calmness they don't want.

Here are some of the ways government, backed by selected civic groups, has used massive resources in attempting to limit the way Americans can use the Internet to enhance their sexual expression, education, or health:

- 1993: Government entraps Californians Robert and Carleen Thomas, operators of a bulletin board and porn distribution company. Postal Inspector David Dirmeyer orders adult material from a Memphis, Tennessee, address and then has them arrested for distribution of obscene material on the Internet. The Court of Appeals, 6th circuit, upholds the conviction in 1996.[30]
- 1995: Congress proposes (but doesn't pass) S.892, the Protection of Children from Computer Pornography Act.
- 1996: Congress passes the Communications Decency Act (CDA), criminalizing sending anything "harmful to minors" over the Internet (overturned in 1997).
- 1996: Senators Hatch (R-UT) and Feinstein (D-CA) cosponsor a law criminalizing the use of "morphing" technology (as opposed to actual children) to create computer images that imitate child porn.
- 1998: Congress passes the Child Online Protection Act. This establishes the Commission on Online Child Protection, and requires *all* commercial distributors of "material harmful to minors" to prevent minors from accessing their Web sites. "Material harmful to minors" is a much lower standard than "obscenity," and includes female breasts.
- 1999: Court of Appeals upholds injunction against enforcing COPA. The government appeals.
- 2000: Congress passes the Child Internet Protection Act, after both CDA and COPA are overturned.[31] This requires libraries and schools receiving federal funds to install filtering software on their computers.
- 2000–2005: various state governments pass "mini-COPAs," criminalizing the use of the Internet to send anything "harmful to minors." These laws are generally overturned by the courts.[32]
- 2000–present: Various states establish that those repairing others' computers, whether employed in the same company or in business as

repair shops, are mandated reporters of suspected child pornography—without any training in evaluating this material or protection for those inappropriately reported.

- 2002: Attorney General Ashcroft announces a new "war on porn."
- 2003: The Supreme Court upholds CIPA, establishing the constitutionality of requiring mandatory filtering of legal material.
- 2003: The Court of Appeals again rules COPA unconstitutional. The government appeals again.
- 2004: The Supreme Court upholds block on enforcement of COPA. The government continues looking for ways to enforce it.
- 2005: The Department of Justice (DOJ) changes the definition of the 2257[33] Regulations, creating extraordinary recordkeeping requirements on all Web sites showing any sexual content. The requirements are retroactive, punitive, clearly not aimed to accomplish their alleged intention (to prevent minors from performing in adult films, and to give government redundant power to punish child pornography). The law is passed despite clear evidence that minors are not performing in contemporary adult films.
- 2005: The Free Speech Coalition sues the DOJ to enjoin the 2257 Regulations until they can be challenged in whole in court.
- 2005: Utah is the latest of 15 states passing Internet censorship laws.[34]
- 2005: Attorney General Gonzales announces a war on obscenity, and creates a porn task force in the Federal Bureau of Investigations.
- 2005: The owners of Web sites (e.g., www.RedRose.com, www.ShadesBeyondGray.com) with sexually explicit words, rather than pictures, are arrested, their Web sites shut down as "obscene." Many well-known fetish Web site publishers self-censor or shut down completely to avoid prosecution (e.g., www.BeautyBound.com, www.KinkyGurl.com, www.RealBDSM.com).
- 2006: The DOJ subpoenas Google, Yahoo!, and MSN to obtain one million random Web addresses and records of all searches for a week as part of trying to get COPA upheld on appeal. The DOJ allegedly does this to prove that blocking and filtering technology doesn't effectively stop children from reaching pornographic Web sites.
- 2008: State governments begin to prosecute minors involved in "sexting" cases.

NEW INTERNET "CRIMES"

By 2008, two new "crimes" had been added to the menu of Internet treachery—(1) sexting by minors and (2) responding to government-sponsored chatroom stings. They both involved the use of imagination to create unauthorized sexual arousal.

Sexting started spontaneously between owners of the powerful new generation of mobile phones, who suddenly had high-quality cameras with them every day—which needed no film, and therefore no film processing by nosy strangers. Like adults, minors started taking sexy pictures of themselves or each other, sending them to boyfriends, girlfriends, or groups of people. Law enforcement officials across the country immediately labeled this activity as distribution of child porn, and threatened that those who were caught would be arrested and even jailed—which is exactly what happened.

Despite predictions that sexting will invite sexual assault and ruin lives, no one has proven that sexting does any real harm. Ten years from now, everyone applying to Harvard Medical School or Stanford Law School will have nude pictures of themselves on the Internet, and perspective employers of these young people will just shrug. It's similar to tattoos 15 years ago—people predicted that those getting inked would regret their indelible choice as they lost out on jobs (and quality mates). Now you can't find a gynecologist or CPA without one.

The real issue with sexting is the regulation of teen sexuality. The War on Sex—already withholding medical and contraceptive information and supplies from teens, already criminalizing a wide range of teen sexual behavior—has now organized this latest attempt to colonize the bodies of America's teens.

The only danger of sexting is the criminal prosecution by authorities attempting to discourage what they claim is a dangerous activity. Phillip Alpert, for example, was 18 in 2009 when he sent a naked photo of his 16-year-old girlfriend (which she had taken and sent him) to dozens of her friends and family after an argument. He was arrested, charged with sending child pornography, sentenced to five years probation, and required to register as a sex offender. As a registered offender, he was thrown out of college, and can't get a job. He's forced to live with his parents—but if they live too close to a school or park, he won't even be able to live with them. His life is completely ruined—a casualty of the War on Sex.[35]

"There are hundreds, if not thousands, of these kids on the sex registration lists across the U.S.," defense attorney Larry Walters says, shaking his head.

The second new Internet "crime" involves going to an adult chatroom, being approached by someone pretending to be a teen, and playing along—until the purported teen is revealed as a police detective, and the unsuspecting "criminal" is charged with being interested in sex with a minor. If the chatroom is reserved for adults, and the detective is an adult, one wonders exactly how this can be anything other than a thought crime. The police reasoning seems to be "Yes, you were texting with an adult cop, but you thought it was a kid, and were planning to do something with her that would be illegal." Claims of "I knew it was an adult, but I was enjoying the game" typically fall on deaf ears—because no busted guy can prove he believed he was talking with an adult.

There's a terribly corrupt angle to this that most Americans don't appreciate. First, federal money (along with paid trips to training seminars) is driving local police departments to set up these stings. The more guys they can entice into communicating with a cop posing as a teen, the more money their department is awarded—a motivational system that's been rejected regarding traffic violations (speed traps, red-light cameras, etc.) and other parts of police work.

Second, the private Internet-monitoring group Perverted Justice has been getting $100,000 per body that they can lure onto NBC's *To Catch a Predator*, the popular "reality" TV program that shows unsuspecting losers walking into stings and collapsing with guilt and shame. As attorney Steve Turer describes, "It's a media-run police action," where the police have subcontracted their authority to a vigilante group that isn't constrained by the same ethics or policies of the police themselves.

Turer's client Joseph Roisman, a young sailor entrapped and busted on national TV in 2006—and acquitted in 2011—is a good example of this repulsive new system that prowls the Internet for men who seem *capable* of having sex with minors. The judge in his Northern California case was so disgusted he threw the case out without even letting a jury vote on it.[36]

SUMMARY

Rather than deal with their fear, rather than recognize the radical potential of the Internet to help fulfill the American promise, those who fear sex have gone the other way—demonizing the Internet, attempting to limit its growth and availability. And they have done this even as they use that same Internet as a tool to undermine the American promises of fact-based public policy, free access to information, and the cherished right to be left alone.

The sad thing is that Americans today must look to the courts to decide that such restrictions are unconstitutional, rather than expecting our elected representatives to say, "No, revoking Americans' freedoms for *any* reason is just not a wise idea—and it is simply not acceptable."

Because the Internet is pure information, it confronts us with a choice that has become far too common, and is even more stark than usual: Which is more dangerous—information, or the consequences of restricting it?

Online predators do pose a threat to a very small number of minors. But revoking even a part of the freedom of 200 million Americans, young and old, is a tangible, meaningful threat that should be preceded by a serious, complex social dialogue. That dialogue *must* include the voices of scientists, sexologists, and those who realize that protecting every single child from every potential harm is simply impossible. And it must respect the stubborn, experienced voices of those who know that without real freedom, safety is an illusion.

Chapter Eleven

AMERICA DOES NOT GUARANTEE YOUR RIGHT TO BE COMFORTABLE: THE LOWEST COMMON EROTIC DENOMINATOR PROJECT

Across America, pictures are coming down and sculpture is being covered; workplaces are being sanitized, as bulletin boards and screen savers are cleared, and e-mail blocking is ever-stricter. College campuses are in the grip of speech codes, as professors are being disciplined for discussing the realities of historical or contemporary gender, intimacy, and, most of all, sexuality.

Now that American culture has decided that sex is a primary source of most of its problems,[1] removing it from the public arena as much as possible is seen as the solution.

The War on Sex is committed to eliminating any public experience that causes *anyone* discomfort around sexuality. This is the Lowest Common Erotic Denominator project. It's stripping us of meaningful art, diminishing our creativity at work, interfering with normal adult relationships, and constraining academic and media discussions of philosophy, social science, the humanities, and politics. But many people apparently feel this is a small price to pay for making sure no one is offended or uncomfortable about sex.

When America outlawed the creation of a "hostile work environment" in the 1980s, the idea was to prevent racial and gender harassment that was repeated, pervasive, and so severe as to obstruct individuals from performing their job.

But now even the most indirect reference to sexuality at work or school can be considered the creation of a hostile employment or learning environment. Given the breadth of sexual influences and expression in human life, this means that any individual can exercise a veto over a huge range of workplace or school issues: dress, language, decor, personal memorabilia, charitable policies, even after-hours recreation. "Hostile environment" law has been perverted to create a right *to not be offended* when one leaves one's home.

While everyone deserves a fair chance to succeed, appealing to the most erotophobic sentiment to create a sexless work or university environment is not about fairness—it's about bleaching eroticism out of society. *This* is patently unfair, and *this* is offensive to many. But sex-positive feelings have no legal standing because people comfortable with sex are not a protected class like ethnic minorities or women. When can someone sue because short skirts are banned in a private office? Or because a gold cross around someone's neck is acceptable, while a silver vulva isn't?

Patrons of public facilities have also acquired the phony "right" to never be uncomfortable about sexuality, no matter how repressed they are about it. This is used to justify Internet filtering in libraries. People applying for driver licenses or phone service are complaining if municipal clerks show too much cleavage. Art that has civilized, comforted, challenged, and enlightened people for 500 years is being taken down from city halls across America.

So whose standard of discomfort shall we use—the person whose threshold of discomfort is lowest? No one says to an employer or city government, "By the way, I'm cool with the thought-provoking artwork around here." No one says, "By the way, I'm fine that the person at the next desk, or the clerk who processed my forms, wears an open marriage button on her lapel."

Those *not* offended by sexual words or images are a crucial part of the continuum of the public's values. But the standards and feelings of those *not* obsessed with sex are never taken seriously in this matter.

Historically, democratic countries have focused primarily on controlling behavior, while totalitarian governments have attempted to control speech and thought as well. American laws of the last 20 years are changing that, however. Public art, company e-mail, and casual speech are increasingly monitored and restricted, as the "feelings" of coworkers, classmates, customers, and neighbors are seen as sufficient reason for government intervention.

Removing a perfectly legal statue or classical play from public view because its sexual aspects make someone *uncomfortable* is increasingly common. The workplace, college campus, and public square are now places where some are entitled to the comfort of not having their sensibilities challenged, while the rest of us suffer arbitrary censorship. In such an inhibited, anxious environment, no one grows, and ultimately everyone loses.

We need laws protecting the rights of people offended by the neurotic stripping of human eroticism from workplaces and civic spaces across America.

Wrestling with eroticism has been one of humanity's most glorious, productive (albeit troubling) challenges throughout history. Every culture that interrupts this adult project pays for it in violence or stagnation; that's the lesson of the Spanish Inquisition, Sharia law, the Soviet Union, and "modern" Iran.

It's no coincidence that in 2002, Attorney General John Ashcroft covered the breast on the 70-year-old "The Spirit of Justice" statue before launching a massive assault on Americans' liberty.

The War on Sex Comes to Campus[a]

Ironically, the bizarre American concept that people deserve protection from unwanted or uncomfortable sexual feelings (as opposed to a *pervasive, ongoing, hostile* environment that prevents normal learning or working) has reached its peak in America's colleges—the place where (1) the exchange of ideas is supposed to be most open and rewarding, and (2) young adults learn to tolerate a wide range of people and emotional challenges.

Intellectual exchange and the protection of feelings, of course, are fundamentally at odds; driven by the religion-morality group-conservative feminist apparatus of the War on Sex, academia today sacrifices the first on the altar of the second. Unfortunately, this decade-long trend was recently supercharged by the government, and by the predictable response of the attorneys for the country's colleges.

On April 4, 2011, the federal Department of Education's Office for Civil Rights (OCR) issued a dramatic 19-page letter[b] detailing procedures every university must follow in cases of alleged sexual harassment or sexual assault. A college that fails to follow these guidelines risks the possibly devastating loss of federal funding—Yale, for example, could lose half a billion dollars.

The fact that "sexual harassment" (which is primarily about feelings) and "sexual assault" (which is supposed to be about physical experiences) are covered in the same document by similar rules is the first clue of dangerous policy implications.

Most university sexual harassment policies include campus speech codes—policies that restrict speech typically protected by the First Amendment off campus (also known as "the real world"). Suddenly, student breaches of these repressive speech codes were potentially the cause for dramatic losses by colleges.

Worse, in these sexually oriented cases, the OCR now demands that colleges lower their standards of justice, adopting a "preponderance of the evidence" (i.e., a 50.01%, or "more likely than not") standard of proof—far lower than an accused is supposed to receive in a normal trial in any town in America.

The result—supported by academia's emerging sex-negative traditions and ideologues who want to enforce political correctness—has been to fashion campus procedures that make sexual words, gestures, and even consensual behavior highly dangerous. What people consider normal mating and relationship trial-and-error in town is now enough to get you thrown out of school, your career damaged or destroyed by the black mark of "sexual harasser."

Such policies collapse the distinction between intention, feelings, and behavior, rendering the concept of consent meaningless. These policies infantilize students, making it clear that sexuality (words, feelings, negotiation, emotional conflict) is something against which they need special protection. And the policies empower colleges to deal with sexuality on their own arbitrary terms, establishing sex as a human focus that requires special intervention.

This is a corruption of the university-student relationship, and the destruction of any presumption of trust or communication between students. Frank discussions about sexual behavior or identity are off-limits on such campuses. Flirting and the gauging of another's interest can no longer be innocent or merely sporting. And these speech codes give virtually anyone on campus a tool with which to punish virtually anyone else on campus. That's particularly true of the administration—which can punish almost any student it wishes if he or she is a troublemaker, or offends someone powerful.

In 2010, FIRE, a non-partisan non-profit that defends free speech on college campuses, found that 67% of the 390 colleges it surveyed maintain policies "that are laughably unconstitutional under First Amendment standards."[c]

Keeping in mind that being accused of sexual harassment or of violating a speech code means your rights of due process are unusually slender for the American justice system, here are some examples of what now constitutes sexual harassment according to the current policies at various colleges across the country:

- California State University–Monterey Bay: "may range from sexual innuendoes made at inappropriate times, perhaps in the guise of humor, to coerced sexual relations"
- Alabama State University: "behavior that causes discomfort, embarrassment or emotional distress"
- University of Iowa: something that "occurs when somebody says or does something sexually related that you don't want them to say or do, regardless of who it is"

- Iowa State University: "can range from unwelcome sexual flirtations and inappropriate put-downs of individual persons or classes of people to serious physical abuses such as sexual assault"
- San Francisco State University: "one person's distortion of a university relationship by unwelcome conduct which emphasizes another person's sexuality"
- Murray State University: "elevator eyes"
- Davidson College: "innuendoes, teasing, jokes, derogatory or dismissive comments; starting or spreading rumors; whistling, hooting, growling, lip smacking, kissing noises" and "wearing inappropriate or sexually suggestive clothing"
- University of California–Berkeley: "humor and jokes about sex in general that make someone feel uncomfortable"
- Bryn Mawr College: "slang names, or labels that others could find offensive."
- Columbia University: "love letters"
- Yale University: "unspoken sexual innuendo, such as voice inflection when complimenting appearance"
- University of California—Santa Cruz: "terms of endearment"
- Drexel University: "holding or eating food provocatively"

In addition, many college policies attempt to control the actual consensual sexual practices of students. For example, Yale encourages students to "communicate verbally before engaging in sexual activity." The policy also requires that "consent must be clear and unambiguous for each participant at every stage of a sexual encounter." This policy was apparently crafted by someone who has never heard of mood, chemistry, instinct, sensuality, cooperation, or trust. "Unambiguous?" The majority of college students—and of adults in general—are not nearly so unambivalent about sexuality that they can rise to such a standard.

Grambling State University's policy is simpler, if far more ridiculous and flatly unconstitutional: "all consensual sexual activity and/or sexual intercourse (copulation) on the University premises is strictly prohibited." Nice way to teach adults how to think, communicate, and negotiate. And to be honest about what they're doing.

[a]With special appreciation to the Foundation for Individual Rights in Education and its president, Greg Lukianoff (see www.thefire.org).
[b]http://thefire.org/article/13143.html.
[c]http://www.huffingtonpost.com/greg-lukianoff/yale-the-department-of-ed_b_877467.html.

Chapter Twelve

BATTLEGROUND: THE WAR ON "PORNOGRAPHY"

When Attorney General Alberto Gonzales announced the new federal war on pornography in 2005, with increased funding and reassignment of eight full-time FBI agents, one law enforcement veteran snidely expressed what a lot of people were thinking: "I guess we've won the war on terror."[1]

We hadn't, of course, so here's a clue to the real payoff: According to the *Washington Post*, "Christian conservatives, long skeptical of Gonzales, greeted the pornography initiative with what the Family Research Council called 'a growing sense of confidence in our new Attorney General.' "[2]

Prosecuting pornography was a political bone. The Bush administration, wanting to burnish the conservative credentials of its lagging Justice Department, threw the bone to the Right, which eagerly leaped for it.

Acquiring the support of the Family Research Council in exchange for simply limiting every American's right to private entertainment must have seemed like a terrific deal to the Bush administration. Their war on porn was no more about making America's families safer than was Ronald Reagan's Meese Commission 20 years before it.

But restricting the amount and type of sexually explicit material you're allowed to look at in private (and attempting to drive its producers and distributors out of business) is only one part of the battle against pornography. The other is a massive disinformation campaign—some of it sincere, much of it manipulative, and too much of it outright lies. This campaign has seduced, in no particular order, journalists, feminists, safety advocates, liberals—even small-government conservatives.

We're not talking about porn that involves kids. No professional pornographer, no progressive sexologist, no libertarian, no sane person advocates involving actual children in the creation of pornography. Let's agree this is *not* under discussion, and proceed.

Well, it would be nice if we could do that. Unfortunately, anti-porn activists focus obsessively on the alleged connection between adult porn and child porn, making an intelligent conversation difficult. As we'll see later, there is no connection between the two.

In addition, anti-porn activists are obsessed with so-called "violent porn"—a heterogeneous category that mostly includes on-screen characters having fun playing with dominance and submission. Some of your neighbors play these sexual games, involving pain, surrender, intensity—and trust. Their faces may grimace, and their voices cry out, their bodies may look contorted or tormented. But millions of adults play like this, and so actors and actresses sometimes portray these games.

Screen characters can also portray violent, coercive behavior—some of it in porn films. Porn or not, most viewers know that the actors in these films are working under carefully controlled conditions—after all, it's just a movie. And porn or not, extremely violent films are a sub-genre with limited appeal. Actually, a far larger percentage of mainstream films depict extreme violence than the percentage of porn films that depict extreme violence.

Both illegal child porn and legal extremely violent porn represent a tiny minority of the pornography that's actually available and consumed by America's 50 million porn viewers.

That leaves the rest of porn, in which actors portray happy male and female characters doing things they enjoy. Sometimes their fun involves stuff you find pleasurable that someone else might not: oral sex, spanking, anal toys, whatever. Occasionally these characters pursue activities you or your mate might *not* want to do: exhibitionism, playing with urine, group sex, whatever. Either way, *the overwhelming majority of porn portrays consenting, enthusiastic men and women doing things they enjoy.* These are activities routinely indulged in by tens of millions of Americans, *sexual activities that couples go to marriage counselors to get more comfortable with.*

So when a discussion about porn turns to "extremely violent porn" or "kiddie porn" or "bestiality," these are not representative of mainstream adult material. Condemning all porn because of these exotic subgenres is like eliminating all TV because *The Three Stooges* is stupid or *The Sopranos* is violent. When you hear or participate in a conversation about pornography, see if the other person can talk without referring to porn "addiction," child porn, brutal porn, or mass murder. If they can't, they're not discussing pornography, or even sex; they're discussing violence, power, sadism, and fear.

And the extremely violent porn that a tiny sliver of consumers enjoys? It is disturbing that some people get pleasure or relief from watching such images. But it isn't a reminder that porn is bad. It's a reminder that human sexuality—like human psychology in general—is complex, some of it quite dark. Our society hasn't come to terms with this, and so it wars on the material that supposedly creates this darkness. That's willfully naïve. Every society has people who resonate with violent imagery, whether it's a porn film, a bullfight, Indy car crashes, or the experience of war. Fortunately, most people who resonate with violent porn (or bullfights, or other violent imagery) don't act out their response.

A WAR ON PEOPLE

The war on porn is a war on people—people who look at porn. The government and conservative groups talk about "pornographers" and "hardcore smut," but rarely about consumers of adult pornography—which total some 50 million Americans. To put that in perspective, *The Daily Show* gets about 2 million viewers in a typical week, and David Letterman gets about 4 million. About 30 million Americans have seen a Harry Potter film in a theater.

Clearly, adult pornography is mainstream entertainment. And obviously, all its 50 million viewers aren't "porn addicts," psychopaths, or child molesters. But claiming they are opens the door for a wide range of attacks on pornography. For many people, this public attacking behavior is driven by private emotional issues.

Americans are anxious about their sexual "normality" and competence, and about the impact of modern life on their relationships and their kids. Many of us are taught to feel guilty about our sexual desires, fantasies, and bodies, and this shame leads to secrecy, which complicates things. There may be no easy answers, but people still want their anxiety and emotional isolation to go away.

We want our kids to be sexually healthy, but we don't know how to talk with them—and the sexualized media scare us. We want our sexual relationships to be enjoyable and nourishing, but we don't know how to talk with our mates, and what we're told about everyone else's sex lives scares us.

In this context of emotional vulnerability, people welcome simple explanations that identify clear villains and provide clear solutions. The clergy, our government, the media, feminist groups, and "morality groups" insist that porn is the villain, and fighting porn is the answer. You've observed that many

Americans love this. People in pain love knowing that there's a "them" to blame and an "it" to attack.

The war on porn is a psychologically perfect solution to the confusion, anger, self-criticism, and shame that many Americans feel about sexuality and modern life. It's short-sighted, futile, self-destructive, undignified, and disempowering. But it provides an explanation, a target, and hope. *It's a public policy solution to a private emotional problem.* And it empowers and emboldens leaders and institutions who manipulate the public into thinking that sexuality is the *problem*, when sexual self-acceptance, flexibility, skills, and knowledge are the *answer.*

The war on pornography is also a handy activity for people who *use* porn and feel ashamed, guilty, and afraid of God's judgment. Like anti-prostitution crusaders who see hookers, or anti-gay activists found in gay bars, many anti-porn advocates are simply trying to distance themselves from their own impulses. These people deserve sympathy, not a place at the public policy table.

Pornography is the repository of our culture's ambivalence and negativity about sex (e.g., Americans watch porn, but pretend they don't. They masturbate, but pretend they don't).

Porn contains, for the most part, portrayals of conventional (many would say "normal") sex—intercourse, oral sex, masturbation, orgasm, vibrators, anal sex, power games. Nevertheless, our society damns these portrayals—which are the *record of,* and therefore the *acknowledgement of,* our fantasy, desire, and participation. Porn is the opposite of the closet, of our culture's shame about sexuality. And so those who speak from ambivalence or negativity angrily confront those who use porn: "It's bad enough that you enjoy lusty sex. If you can't have the decency to feel guilty about your sexuality, you certainly don't have to celebrate it, much less deliberately inflame your desire!"

It's not simply that so many of us are uncomfortable about sexuality. *It's the relationship that individuals and the culture have with that discomfort.* The discomfort does not get discussed honestly, nor do most people feel in any way obligated to resolve these feelings. Instead, the discomfort is considered normal and fixed, and the objects of the discomfort—pornography, along with sexual words, music, art, and expression—are considered "bad" and expendable.

This is one reason that pornography is demonized. People want to conceptualize and describe it as being far enough away from what's "normal" so that there's no question about which has to change—the *objects* of the discomfort, not the discomfort *itself.* The demonization of pornography is a way of ending any dialogue before it really starts. If you defend or even accept pornography, you're saying the equivalent of "I'm selfish, ignorant, misogynist, and perverted."

There should be room in America's ongoing discourse for discussing people's pain about pornography, and our concern about some of our neighbors' usage of it. But it is unacceptable to make that the *only* conversation about pornography. The government has taken that position strongly, which is cynical, dishonest, and destructive. It would be like making anorexia and bulimia the center of every discussion about nutrition or weight control.

To put it another way, if all we have is the wrong conversation about pornography, we end up eliminating a lot of sexual expression, at a social, psychological, and constitutional cost that's unacceptable. It's the equivalent of burning down a house to fumigate it.

THE WAR ON PORN

Here are some of the ways government and anti-porn forces are warring on pornography *and those who view it*.

- Limiting what can be downloaded from/uploaded to the Internet, and what can be e-mailed. The federal government has been attempting to legislate this since 1996; Pennsylvania, Arizona, New York, and Michigan have also tried (and were defeated in federal court). In 2010, a federal court blocked[3] a new Massachusetts statute that, incredibly, criminalized sending anything over the Internet into the state that might be "harmful to minors," even if it was legal for adults to see it. Limiting sales of popular magazines (including *Cosmopolitan* and *Glamour)* in convenience stores and supermarkets. The nation's 7–Elevens stopped selling *Playboy, Penthouse*, and other soft-core magazines in 1986 when the federal Meese Commission threatened to list the parent Southland Corporation (and two dozen other convenience store chains) as a "distributor of pornography" in its report. Although the threat was clearly illegal (and was declared so by a federal judge), the censorship was accomplished.[4]

  Another approach to the sale of legal adult magazines comes from pro-censorship "feminists," such as Melissa Farley. In 1985, she began a National Rampage Against Penthouse with colleague Nikki Craft, which was a campaign of public destruction of bookstore-owned copies of *Penthouse* and *Hustler*. Farley was arrested 13 different times in 9 different states for these actions.[5]

  In September 2011, Dr. Calum Bennachie filed a complaint against Farley with the American Psychiatric Association, asking that her membership be revoked due to numerous alleged violations of ethical research standards and misrepresentation of data.[6]

  Today, local groups periodically picket stores that sell porn magazines or DVDs. They often photograph patrons or their license plates to

discourage them from entering. In 2006, a campaign like this was insti-
gated by actor Stephen Baldwin in Nyack, New York. The American
Family Association's Web site even has instructions on how to do this,
including suggested messages on picket signs.[7]

- Internet filtering—now mandatory for public libraries that want
  federal funds; encouraged by nervous lawyers in universities, hospitals,
  businesses, and other institutions; demanded by "morality groups"
  afraid of sexual information; and marketed to parents across the
  United States concerned about Internet predators and the destructive
  power of certain magic syllables (called by sophisticated people "the F
  word") or a naked female breast. For more on this, see Chapter 10.
- Expanding the definition of "obscenity" to criminalize more depictions and activities—despite the demonstrable fact that American
  sexual mores have become looser and more inclusive. Just try to imagine *South Park, Desperate Housewives*, or *The Sopranos* on your TV in
  1985. Remember how startling *NYPD Blue* was only 15 years ago?
- Expecting computer repair shops, photo developing shops, and other
  businesses to report "suspicious" material to police. Not surprisingly,
  grandmothers have been arrested for bathtub photos of their grand-
  children, and computers have been confiscated by untrained people.

  Tamie Dragone, for example, was detained by police in Salina,
  Kansas, when a Wal-Mart photo clerk decided a semi-nude photo
  she took of her three-year-old was suspicious. Teresa and Charlie
  Hanraty were jailed in Raleigh, North Carolina, over a photo of him
  kissing their baby's naval; they lost custody of their two children.
  And in Portsmouth, New Hampshire, in a single month, not one
  but two computer shops called law enforcement over alleged child
  porn. After examining the owners' private property—no warrant necessary—the computers, and owners, were cleared.
- Demanding that pay-for-porn channels be removed from hotel room
  televisions. In 2000, the Omni hotel chain discontinued in-room
  porn, and in 2002, several Cincinnati hotels, including the Marriott,
  withdrew their adult movies. The domestic erotic terror group Citizens for Community Values then organized a coalition demanding
  that the Justice Department eliminate all hotel porn in the United
  States.
- Pressuring Visa and MasterCard to stop accepting payments from
  porn transactions.
- 2257 Regulations, which require that anyone who exhibits sexually
  explicit pictures, even of performers who are elderly or deceased, be
  able to prove that each performer is over 18. This is an outrageous
  (and incredibly expensive, when you read the regs) "guilty until

proven innocent" intrusion into a legal business operation. Besides, when we're assured that it won't be applied to Broadway or Hollywood productions, doesn't that make it discriminatory and unconstitutional?

- Using zoning laws to eliminate places where stores that sell porn or offer video booths can legally operate.
- Congressional hearings that start with the assumption that pornography is bad for individuals and society. Testimony from anti-porn ideologues and "morality" groups is solicited to validate this view; sexologists, social scientists, and consumers are specifically excluded from testifying.
- The invention of "porn addiction," which was a logical extension of the invention of "sex addiction," by prison addictionologist Patrick Carnes. Various psychologists, clergy, and "morality leaders" claim that men become addicted to porn and have to be cured by discontinuing use altogether. Many expensive treatment programs even insist that "sobriety" means no masturbation whatsoever.
- Establishing "Victims of Pornography Month" (each May). President George W. Bush himself endorsed this, saying that "pornography is now instantly available to any child who has a computer. And in the hands of incredibly wicked people, the Internet is a tool that lures children into real danger." And the relevance of this to adult porn creation and use is . . . what?[8]
- The myth of activist judges: The idea that porn could be limited or banned "if only" certain judges would stop "creating" law to tolerate porn. This completely misses the point that America has two centuries of laws protecting free expression (even if it offends someone), which judges are supposed to enforce when legislators or police break them. The Traditional Values Coalition even has a "battle plan to take back the courts from the ACLU and the anti-God Left."[9] They conveniently forget the large number of sitting judges who were appointed by Republicans.
- Most of the public doesn't realize that their marriage counselor, psychologist, physician, social worker, clergymember or other clinician probably received absolutely no training in the realities of adult entertainment. Without training, these clinicians can only fall back on the anti-porn myths saturating the media and their professions' sex-negative traditions. Unfortunately, many professionals believe that being trained to treat "porn addiction" is the same as learning about porn use in the general population.
- When the government decides to bust a store that sells adult material, it typically seizes most or even all of the store's inventory so that the

defendant can't pay the legal costs of fighting the arrest. Remember, authorities cannot simply declare an inventory obscene—that is, potentially illegal. Only a jury can do that.[10]

• Establishing porn taxes: singling out sexually oriented products for special, very high (typically 10 to 25%) taxes. Enabling legislation has been proposed in at least a half-dozen states, including California in 2008 and New York and Washington in 2009. A federal porn tax bill was introduced by Senator Blanche Lincoln (D-AR) in 2005, co-sponsored by nine Democrats. It couldn't get through the Republican-controlled Senate.[11]

WHAT ABOUT KIDDIE PORN?

The American porn industry neither makes nor distributes erotic material knowingly featuring underage performers. Anyone who says otherwise is a liar and should be asked to provide proof. The War on Sex is full of liars who raise blood pressures—and millions of tax-deductible dollars—lying about this.

The underage material available in the U.S. today is either (1) amateur stuff made by individuals and distributed surreptitiously or (2) made by foreign producers in Russia, Eastern Europe, and Asia, with no affiliation to American businesses. Thus, further regulating the American adult industry will have *no effect whatsoever* on the amount of underage porn available in the United States. It may make legislators look good and constituents feel good, but it will not decrease the availability of, nor the appetite for, the material that everyone agrees is illegal and unconscionable.

In fact, in 1996, the American adult industry established the Association of Sites Advocating Child Protection (ASACP), a nonprofit organization dedicated to eliminating child pornography from the Internet. ASACP's efforts include a reporting hotline for Web surfers and Web masters, rewards for accurate reporting/conviction of those responsible for child porn, strict standards for American adult Web sites, and proactive educational campaigns about age verification and other topics. During its existence, ASACP has received over a half-million reports of suspected child pornography sites. Virtually all (99.9%) of these reports can be attributed to non-adult Web masters, amateur collectors, or pedophiles, not professional adult companies.[12]

Given today's political and economic realities, no one could be more interested in the elimination of child porn than the U.S. adult industry. It is fascinating to observe how the most ridiculous rumors to the contrary are so persistent, for example, that porn is marketed to children. Since children have no credit cards with which to purchase porn, why on earth would marketing target them?

Anti-porn activists also consistently spread the falsehood that watching adult porn leads to desiring and watching kiddie porn. If this is true, how do activists explain the following?

- The overwhelming majority of adult porn consumers do *not* consume child porn.
- The majority of child porn consumers are not regular consumers of adult porn.

Activists point to the fact that some men caught with child pornography also consume adult pornography. Of course they do. If you take any random 1,000 male customers of United Airlines or Hertz Car Rentals, you'd discover that a large percentage of them consume adult pornography as well.

Is America soft on kiddie porn? Hardly. Current federal law criminalizes:

- Any depictions of minors being sexual with another person, adult or minor
- Any sexually oriented depictions of adults who *appear* to be minors
- Any sexuality-oriented artificial or digitally created images that *appear* to be of minors
- Falsely *advertising* that a sexually oriented image of an adult is actually of a minor
- And the perfect catch-all category, any "lascivious exhibition of the genital area" of a minor—which can mean, say, photos of fully-clothed young teens, babies, or other minors if a jury decides the camera has a leering gaze

This is, of course, in addition to the completely redundant, totally symbolic (and expedient for the politicians who passed them) child pornography laws in each of the 50 states.

And if you think this legislative overkill is insufficient, you'll love House Bill 1981, which came out of committee on July 28, 2011. Called the Protecting Children From Internet Pornographers Act of 2011 (which is an immediate tipoff that it's about the politics of moral panic, not actual protection), it requires every Internet service provider to track *all of your Internet activity* and save it for 18 months, along with your name, credit card numbers, and the IP addresses you've been assigned. Not because you've done anything wrong, but because this massive intrusion into the personal lives of 100 million Americans *might* catch a handful of traders in child porn. The *Atlantic* calls this mandatory tracking of innocent Americans "arguably the biggest threat to civil liberties now under consideration in the United States."[13] The

Electronic Frontier Foundation calls the bill "ripe for abuse by law enforcement officials," creating "a perfect storm for government abuse."

THE PUBLIC HEALTH MODEL—A CLEVER MANIPULATION

Those who wish to limit or ban pornography have cleverly positioned it (and thus, fighting it) as a public health issue. We hear, for example, about its supposed co-morbidities (fear of intimacy, low self-esteem, perversion); supposed effects on consumers (addiction, depression, isolation, disrespect for women); supposed impact on communities (increased violence, divorce, tumbling morals)—and the ultimate health issue, that it's supposedly bad for kids.[14]

It's a familiar model, generally accompanied by a familiar imperative: do what's necessary to clean up the threat and protect our kids and communities, even if it costs a bundle and involves curtailing a few rights. As anthropologist Carole Vance says, "Every right-winger agrees that porn leads to women's inequality—an inequality that doesn't bother him in any other way."[15]

In this context, discussing pornography as a free speech or civil rights issue can sound rather unconvincing and even naïve to many people. In some ways, this reflects a deeper problem with our society; while health and safety problems easily acquire special public policy cachet, many Americans seem to feel that free expression and civil rights are less important than almost anything else under discussion.[16]

For starters, the manipulative, extreme claims of the public health model should be challenged. Instead of apologizing or rolling our eyes, we must loudly say that *science has not shown that adult material causes* these awful consequences. In the same way that coffee often *accompanies* divorce, it's true that many personal and community difficulties *coexist* with adult material. That's because the use of adult material is so widespread, not because it typically causes problems.

And just like there's healthy food and fattening food, safe beaches and beaches dangerous for inexperienced swimmers, there's healthy porn and porn that might not be good for someone. Of course, that depends primarily on the consumer; just like green peppers are hard for a few people to digest and easy for most everyone else, most porn consumers have no trouble "digesting" what they view. The fact that a tiny percentage of viewers have personality disorders is no more reason to banish porn from everyone than the fact that some people can't digest dairy products is good enough reason to remove half-and-half and Häagen-Dazs from supermarkets.

Just like there's such a thing as moderate drinking, there's such a thing as moderate porn use. And while some people can't handle even one or two drinks, most adults can—and they are allowed to. Americans even have the right to drink to excess—as long as they don't behave in dangerous ways. We must challenge the idea that all use of porn is abuse of porn (and therefore hazardous). It isn't.

That said, we should be sympathetic about people's *fear* of porn. The American public of non-porn viewers has been traumatized by repetitive, lurid stories of children molested at psychotic orgies; women raped, enslaved, and trafficked; normal men who become drooling, unproductive idiots; loving families destroyed—all because somebody watched an X-rated DVD. Let's agree that such stories, although untrue, are scary, and that the fear they engender naturally demands action. Let's appreciate the psychological and citizenship skills it would take to resist that demand—from oneself, one's neighbors, or one's civic or religious leaders.

Realistically, only after this can we expect that a conversation about rights will be taken seriously. We must say over and over that we're talking about *our* rights, not just "pornographers' rights"; that *the right to look at porn is directly related to the right to criticize the government, choose your own religion, and raise your kids free of interference*, and how the wrong approach to porn will inevitably undermine everyone's *non-porn* rights. We've already seen this with attempts to censor network TV airings of *Schindler's List* and *Saving Private Ryan*, and with attempts to remove Harry Potter books from public school libraries because of their so-called satanic influence.

In India, people starve while cows roam the streets. It isn't because they think steak is unhealthy, it's because their religion forbids them to kill or consume animals they consider sacred. We may make fun of this. But at least they don't pretend it's a public health issue.

Framing the war on porn as a public health issue makes it easy to drive people to near-hysteria about this alleged epidemic. The government (supported by conservative feminists and the Religious Right) can then deflect attention from *how* it limits porn's alleged bad effects (i.e., how it limits porn), because "nothing's too good for our kids," and "we need to do whatever it takes to secure the health of America."

While this alleged epidemic rages, and frightened, angry people work overtime to keep porn away from our precious children, we should remind ourselves that there is *still* no evidence that seeing pictures of naked smiling people, or depictions of adult sex, or hearing words like "dick" have a harmful effect on children (or adults). Our technologically advanced, research-oriented society studies practically everything that might be risky—from polyester baby blankets to asbestos tile, high-fat meat, flu shots for the elderly, and driving while sleep-deprived. The government and Religious Right refuse to fund objective studies about the effects of pornography use on the general public. They obviously don't trust what the results might be.

Teaching kids to fear sex, to be ashamed of their bodies, to be secretive about masturbation, to believe men and women are from different planets, to focus on avoiding disease instead of creating pleasure and understanding intimacy—every one of these is more dangerous than catching a glimpse of pubic hair. And all of these together—what some people consider normal childrearing—constitute a recipe for heartbreak, dysfunction, and erotic guilt.

PREDICTING MASSIVE CHANGE—A REAL-WORLD EXPERIMENT

Say we had been sitting around in 1999, speculating: "What do you suppose would happen if America was flooded with free, high-quality pornography for a decade?" Many "decency" advocates and danger-oriented feminists would have predicted absolute mayhem: more of every kind of dreadful social pathology, especially sexual violence and relationship disruption.

As it happens, a year later that's the exact experiment America began. The arrival of high-speed broadband Internet into American homes immediately brought mass consumption of pornography. And indeed, the "decency" advocates and erotophobic activists tell us that this level of pornography use has

Figure 12.1.
Effects of Increased Pornography Use

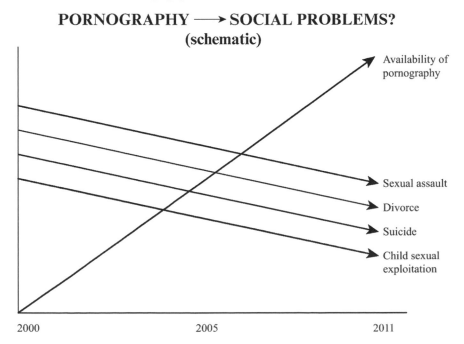

Really—Is Porn Harmful?

The links between pornography and any changes in perceptions, attitudes, and behaviors are circumscribed, few in number and generally laboratory-based.[a]

—*Report of Surgeon General C. Everett Koop, in Ronald Reagan-appointed Meese Commission report*

No evidence of a relationship between popular sex magazines and violence against women.[b]

—*Dr. Cynthia Gentry, Wake Forest University, "Pornography and Rape: An Empirical Analysis"*

There is no systematic research evidence available which suggests a causal relationship between pornography and morality. There is no systematic research which suggests that increases in specific forms of deviant behavior, reflected in crime trend statistics (e.g., rape) are causally related to pornography. There is no persuasive evidence that the viewing of pornography causes harm to the average adult, or that exposure caused the average adult to harm others . . . or that exposure causes the average adult to alter established sex practices.[c]

—*H. B. McKay and D. J. Dolff, "The Impact of Pornography: An Analysis of Research and Summary of Findings"*

In European countries where restrictions on porn have been lifted, incidence of rape over the last 20 years has stayed constant or declined. Between 1965 and 1982, after Denmark made pornography more accessible to the public, sex crimes against female children dropped by 80%.[d]

—*Berl Kutchinsky, "Pornography and Rape: Theory and Practice? Evidence from Crime Data in Four Countries Where Pornography Is Easily Available"*

The aggregate data on rape and other violent or sexual offenses from four countries where pornography, including aggressive varieties, has become widely and easily available during the period we have dealt with would seem to exclude, beyond any reasonable doubt, that this availability has had any detrimental effects in the form of increased sexual violence.[e]

—*Berl Kutchinsky, "Pornography, Sex Crime, and Public Policy"*

Participants exposed to explicit sexual content without accompanying violence did not become desensitized.
>   —*Daniel Linz, Edward Donnerstein, and Steven Adams,*
>   *in* Measuring the Effects of Sexual Content in the Media:
>   A Report to the Kaiser Family Foundation

In West Germany, rape rates declined once bans on pornography were lifted in 1973.
>   —*Philip D. Harvey,* The Government vs. Erotica:
>   The Siege of Adam & Eve

After a three-year inquiry into the effects of pornography, the Committee found that non-violent sexually explicit material does not cause violence or aggression.
>   —*Australian Joint Select Committee on Video Material*

Results from the Czech Republic showed, as seen everywhere else studied (Canada, Croatia, Denmark, Germany, Finland, Hong Kong, Shanghai, Sweden, USA), that rape and other sex crimes have not increased following the legalization and wide availability of pornography.
>   —*Milton Diamond et al. (2010), Pornography and sex crimes in the Czech*
>   *Republic. Archives of Sexual Behavior.* Footnote: DOI 10.1007/
>   s10508-010-9696-y

The amount of pornography a subject used did not predict whether he would hold negative attitudes toward women.
>   —*Alan McKee, Queensland University of Technology, Australia*

The U.S. states with the most internet access have seen twice the decrease in reported rapes as the states with the least internet access.
>   —*Public Law & Legal Theory Research Paper Series,*
>   *Northwestern University*
>   http://anthonydamato.law.northwestern.edu/Adobefiles/porn.pdf

Users of mainstream non-violent pornography in Croatia and non-users felt the same degree of intimacy in their current or recent relationships.
>   —*Archives of Sexual Behavior*

It is certainly clear from the data reviewed that a massive increase in available pornography in Japan has been correlated with a dramatic decrease in sexual crimes, and most so among youngsters as perpetrators or victims—despite the wide increase in availability of pornography to children. Between 1975 and 1995, reported rapes declined by more than half.[f]

—Milton Diamond, "The Effects of Pornography: An International Perspective"

"Sexual abuse *declined* 58% between 1990 and 2008," just as American pornography use was exploding.

—David Finkelhor, Lisa Jones, and Anne Shattuck,
Updated Trends in Child Maltreatment, *2008*[g]

[a]U.S. Department of Justice, Attorney General's Commission on Pornography, by Edwin Meese (Washington, DC: Government Printing Office, 1986).
[b]*Deviant Behavior: An Interdisciplinary Journal* 12 (1991). 277–88.
[c]In Working Papers on Pornography and Prostitution Report No. 3 (Canada: Department of Justice, Canada, in Joint Select Committee Report, 1988).
[d]*International Journal of Law and Psychiatry* 14, no. 1 and 2 (1991): 47–64. (presentation to the Australian Institute of Criminology Conference, "The Sex Industry and Public Policy," Sydney, May 6–8, 1991.)
[e]Aletha C. Huston, Ellen Wartella, and Edward Donnerstein. April 30, 1998. (Amherst, NY: Prometheus Books, 2001), 273
[f]In *Porn 101: Eroticism, Pornography, and the First Amendment*, ed. James Elias et al. (Amherst, NY: Prometheus Books, 1999)
[g]*Published by Crimes Against Children Research Center.*

brought America the very mayhem that they predicted: violence against women, abortion, and a collapse of the country's morals.

The data, however, proves they're wrong.

According to the FBI and other government sources, many leading indicators of social pathology have *declined* since much of the country became regularly involved in pornography (see Figure 12.1). While there's no proof that increased use of pornography has led to these various (and welcome) declines, this data very clearly suggests that pornography use does *not* lead to these negative outcomes, contrary to the constant pronouncements of Morality in Media, Witherspoon Institute, Concerned Women for America, and others promoting today's moral panic.

And by the way, why are all of these groups lying about the supposed ever-increasing amount of sexual violence in America, when the FBI says it's been steadily declining for a decade?

Those who disapprove of pornography insist that it's bad for us. Since neither research nor law enforcement can find any actual data supporting this belief, and so many people watch it without negative effects, the latest "proof" is "brain science," which supposedly shows that porn damages our brain, affecting it like destructive drugs. Purveyors of this junk science include Judith Reisman (discoverer of our self-poisoning "erototoxins"), Marnia Robinson (who claims porn viewing changes men's neurological wiring, leading to chronic erectile dysfunction), and Mary Anne Layden ("Porn addicts have more trouble recovering from their addiction than cocaine addicts").[17]

Serious scientists consistently dismiss this alleged brain data. Of *course* the brain lights up when we look at porn. It also lights up when we look at a Rembrandt, a sunset, or a touchdown pass. Anyone who looks at porn when his or her brain *isn't* lighting up has a *real* problem. And by the way—the actual data behind the claims of junk "neuroscience? As Robinson says, "read the stories on my Web site." In the world of science and fact, we call these *anecdotes*—charming, but not useful.

A NEW GOVERNMENT STRATEGY—FEELING GOOD WHILE ACCOMPLISHING NOTHING

In 1988, the federal government introduced a new law, quickly known as 2257. It required extraordinarily onerous and absolutely unique recordkeeping from the adult industry, with enormous penalties for the most trivial failures to comply. The regulations look exactly like a Soviet-style bureaucratic obstacle to free expression.

Ostensibly to eliminate (non-existent) underage performers from the business, the government demands that anyone producing Web sites, magazines, DVDs, or other sexual material collect and archive photo identification (indexing and cross-referencing every name each performer has ever used) for every nude photo disseminated. "Even if a couple is in their 60s, you have to prove they're over 18," says Robert McGinley, President of Lifestyles Organization. "Since they can't just criminalize all sexy pictures, the government has created a new category of crime involving recordkeeping."

What a sneaky, undignified way around the rights of free expression. While pornography itself can't be criminalized, the government created a way to pursue legal production companies for inadequate recordkeeping. The law was struck down as unconstitutional on First Amendment grounds shortly after its passage.[18] Since then, the discriminatory statute has been resurrected and challenged many times.

In 2005, the government introduced an even stricter new strategy for controlling the production and distribution of legal sexually explicit material. The Department of Justice decided that "secondary producers" (packagers of existing, legal, already-2257-compliant porn) were subject to the same recordkeeping requirements as the original producers. Overnight, hundreds of thousands of Web sites became illegal. A series of court battles ensued, which ended in 2010 with 2257 being upheld.

The 2257 Regulations have been the subject of multiple lawsuits. "The statute imposes heavy burdens on a broad category of protected speech, namely sexually explicit images, based solely on the basis of the content of that speech," wrote the attorneys (including Louis Sirkin and Paul Cambria) who represented the plaintiffs in *Free Speech Coalition v. Gonzales*.[19] The regulations "reach a vast amount of protected speech that not even arguably involves children, and which are outside the Government's interest in controlling child pornography."

The 2257 Regulations pretend to solve a problem that doesn't exist—underage performers in commercial porn—in a way that just happens to create enormous operating burdens for the adult industry. The government shrugs and falls back on a favorite justification: eliminating child porn. Since virtually everyone supports this goal, those who challenge the law look like creeps. Even if that's all 2257 accomplishes, the government wins.

But of course, the logistical nightmare of the regulations will force many smaller producers and distributors out of business (achieving the government's primary, though unstated, goal), and it gives the government the unlimited right to examine and challenge the detailed operations of the rest. During the eight years that the government obsessively stalked retailer Adam & Eve (*PHE, Inc. v. United States Department of Justice*, 1990, *United States v. PHE*, 1992),[20] it admitted that it saw harassment as a legitimate law enforcement tool when porn is involved. 2257 is the latest flavor of harassment.

"The government has the same data as ASACP. They must know that 99.9 percent of child porn has nothing to do with the professional adult industry," says Joan Irvine, ASACP executive director. "The new 2257 rules will not stop the production or distribution of child pornography. Adult companies already comply with the current laws; the criminals involved in child porn don't and never will. I wish the government would focus their time and financial resources on apprehending the real criminals, and truly saving children."[21]

2257 and other attempts to curtail porn use are pointless, says University of California–Los Angeles Law School professor Eugene Volokh. No matter how much the U.S. government can curtail domestic porn distribution, foreign sites will take up the slack. "It's not like Americans have some great irreproducible national skills in smut-making. And even if overall world production of porn somehow improbably falls by 75 percent, will that seriously affect the typical porn consumer's diet? Does it matter whether you have, say, 100,000 porn titles to choose from, or just 25,000? The investment of major prosecutorial resources yields a net practical benefit of roughly zero."

2257 won't change that, but it will create plenty of dangerous constitutional precedents.

Of course the government, continues Volokh, can go after porn consumers. Set up phony sites to entrap American users, then arrest, prosecute, and lock them up. Seize their houses on the theory that it's a forfeitable asset. Make each one register as a sex offender. That would reduce porn consumption. Is America ready to acknowledge what it would take to dramatically change the entertainment habits of one-quarter of the adult population?[22]

WARRING ON PORN AND TERROR

There's an increasing—and creepy—association between America's war on porn and its war on terrorism.

In 2004 and 2005, Chris Wilson operated a Web site from his Florida home, NowThatsFuckedUp.com. It offered pleasant amateur porn (and many discussion groups) for a small fee. One interesting feature was that American soldiers received free entry if they sent photos of themselves from Iraq or Afghanistan. Hundreds did—including grisly war-theatre photos that the government didn't want Americans to see. Remember, this is while the news media were prohibited from showing the coffins of returning American soldiers, as well as battlefield scenes of Iraqi or American casualties.

So Wilson was singled out and busted for obscenity, for hosting a Web site of "free" Americans back home showing off their bodies and having consensual sex in front of the camera. He faced felony charges and 300 misdemeanor counts. He sat in jail two different times, went through two Pentagon investigations (his personal and business computers were shipped to Washington for a forensic examination), and had his home searched.

Facing possible new racketeering (!) forfeiture threats and serious prison time, he plea-bargained. His probation required that he close the site and shun nudity or sex on any future Web site. Wilson and his attorneys agree that the obscenity bust was used to disrupt the soldiers' posting of photos, and to punish Wilson for inviting it.

In early 2006, the Department of Justice asked the four largest Internet search engines in America—Google, AOL, Yahoo!, and MSN—for "a random sample of one million URLs" and the text of every search made over a one-week period.[23] The government wanted the information to help it impose tougher laws on Web sites with information believed to be harmful to minors. Known as "prior restraint," this kind of censorship is prohibited by the U.S. Constitution.

When Google refused to comply, the Department of Justice sought a court order to force them. What gives the government the right to ask for this information? Why, the Patriot Act and other Homeland Security laws—which, an anxious public was told when these laws were passed, were *not* going to be used for precisely this kind of broad domestic surveillance.[24]

But such laws beg to be abused—and unauthorized sexual expression is the perfect vehicle with which the government can abuse them.

So on February 9, 2006, uniformed officers of Montgomery County's Department of Homeland Security marched into a public library in Bethesda, Maryland, and announced that it was forbidden to use library computers to view pornography. They then challenged a patron about the Web site he was visiting and asked him to step outside. A courageous librarian intervened, the police came, and the Homeland defenders had to withdraw, clearly operating outside their authority.[25]

The unannounced, unrecorded "sneak-and-peak" searches of our homes, gadgets, and electronic data that will continue under the Patriot Act (in which the government does *not* have to tell you you're under surveillance) require no prior justification. Our government has a history of feeling politically threatened by a broad range of sexual interests; the sexuality of Martin Luther King, Jr., John Lennon, Emma Goldman, Lenny Bruce, and Paul Robeson, among others, has been investigated.

POLYSEMICITY AND DECIPHERING PORN[26]

Polysemicity is the concept that no text or visual image has only a single meaning. Meaning is supplied by the reader or viewer, and so texts and pictures can have as many meanings as beholders. Said another way, the same thing can mean very different things to different people. In fact, the same experience isn't really the same experience to two different people. And offense is generated in the beholder and directed to the material, not the other way around.[27]

To John, ice cream is a treat to be enjoyed; if he eats it, he's OK. To overweight, self-critical Sam, it's a seductive adversary to be avoided; if he eats it, he's a pig. To Sue, wearing a miniskirt is a desperate bid for attention; to Maria, it's a statement of pride in her looks; to Linda, it's a declaration of independence from her husband; to Joann, it's a way to thumb her nose at the church; to Sarah, it's a way to let men know she's sexually available.

The vast majority of porn's critics (and marriage counselors and porn addiction counselors) say they don't watch or read porn. So how can they know what it portrays, much less how viewers interpret what they see or read? True, porn's critics include a number of self-described ex-porn addicts. Are the reports of these self-described sick, compulsive, spiritually dead, self-destructive people the source of all the anti-porn movement's information?

People who don't view porn (who typically know very little about it) assume that the experience of viewers is the same as the experience a non-viewer would have. It's easy to imagine a non-viewer—say, someone who's never seen two women kissing, or done anal sex, or been ejaculated on, or had sex with the lights on—imagining that looking at porn is uncomfortable, gross, or perverse. It's easy for that person to imagine that anyone acting in such a film is feeling humiliated or being coerced or hurt. And it's easy for that person to imagine that anyone who enjoys looking at porn is emotionally troubled, angry at his wife, or sexually perverse—willing to be violent, coercive, exploitive, or worse.[28]

One reason the concept of "porn addiction" is so appealing is that it explains behavior—"I'm out of control"—that is otherwise hard for nonviewers to understand, or for viewers themselves to fully accept.

Anti-porn forces continually pontificate about porn viewers and the porn viewing experience. They tell us porn viewers are addicted, immature, anti-woman, intimacy-fearing, selfish, gullible, and of course, dangerous to children.

Perhaps these are the qualities *non-viewers* would have *if they* viewed porn. But characterizing America's 50 million porn consumers this way is just nuts. What's even crazier is the way this has become accepted as truth.

THE TRUTHS THAT PORN TELLS

Although pornography is not a love story, it does tell *some* truths. Not literal truths—few of us look like porn actors and actresses—but more philosophical, eternal truths. Politically relevant truths. That's why porn is ultimately subversive, a key reason that it's under siege.

Although American media and culture obsess about sex, most of us live with simplistic, superstitious, anhedonic, fear- and danger-based concepts of eroticism. Many obvious sexual facts are denied, tabooed, and distorted. Examples include: virtually all children masturbate; virtually everyone has sexual interests; most people fantasize sexually (primarily about "inappropriate" partners or activities); and most people are curious about others' bodies and sex lives.

Pornography tells a variety of truths about sex and gender to viewers who decipher what they're seeing (i.e., the vast majority of consumers). These truths are far more important than the surgically enhanced breasts, abnormally big penises, and casual group sex that are staples of the genre (which when taken literally, of course, are misleading). These truths include:

- Anyone can feel (and thus be) sexy.
- Nothing is inherently non-sexual or non-erotic.
- The only rules in sex are arbitrary.
- Many, many people love sex.

- The erotically "nasty" can be life-affirming.
- Even "nice" people enjoy "nasty" fantasies and games.
- Neither intercourse nor orgasm are the center of sexuality.
- Focusing on sexuality for its own sake is legitimate.
- Women and men who feel secure in their dignity and admit that they love sex can enthusiastically submit erotically, because they don't fear judgment (others' or their own).

These truths, of course, defy America's dominant paradigm about sexuality. In the traditional view, external rules are important; body parts are clearly either sexual or non-sexual; "nice" and "nasty" eroticism are clearly distinguishable from each other; different, non-overlapping groups of people indulge in each; and eroticism is dangerous if people don't control their arousal.

Consumers of pornography regularly visit an erotic world quite different than this. The truth that porn tells is that all people have the option of conceptualizing their sexuality any way they like. Social norms regarding age and beauty, religious norms about godly and ungodly sex, personal fears about acceptance, cultural myths about the human body, all of these are ignorable; none are inevitable. Each of us can triumph over the ways social institutions attempt to control our sexual experience.

Ironically, this paradigm of pornography's truths is what sex therapists try to get couples to understand and install in their own lives. These professionals know that the keys to satisfying sexual relationships are self-acceptance and self-empowerment, not losing a few pounds, buying flowers, going away on vacation, or wild positions.

Porn's subtexts of abundance and validation are as responsible for contemporary cultural resistance—that is, the war on porn—as its explicit presentations of sexual activity.

AMATEUR PORNOGRAPHY AS TRUTH

A new way in which pornography tells the truth even more radically is amateur porn, which has exploded via the democratic frenzy of the Internet. Millions of men and women across the globe are now photographing themselves during various sexual activities, uploading these photos onto personal and commercial Web sites, and inviting the entire computerized world to enjoy them.

The world's largest amateur porn site, www.Voyeurweb.com, gets over 4 million unique visits a *day*. Every year, the site receives photos and videos from over 100,000 individuals and couples.[29] And this is just one amateur Web site.

In contrast to most commercial pornography, common features of amateur porn include:

- A wide range of bodies, including ordinary and even conventionally unattractive ones
- A wide range of adult ages, including people conventionally considered way past the prime of their attractiveness or sexuality
- A mostly unproduced physical environment (poor lighting, composition, etc.)
- A heightened sense of mundane reality (shots with unkempt kitchens or kids' toys in the background, scenes filmed in Motel 6, etc.)
- A sense of humor and even parody (these people are having fun!)

The conventional critique of pornography would not predict amateur porn's meteoric popularity. These criticisms assert that the supernatural beauty of actresses is central, that the desultory domination of actress by actor is crucial, that spectacular genital friction is what viewers most envy and desire.

Amateur pornography turns these assumptions upside down. There are no actresses, only real women. These women aren't pretending to be excited, they *are* excited. They aren't flaunting impossibly perfect bodies, they are enjoying their bodies as they are—some of them gorgeous, most of them imperfect, many of them appealing only insofar as they are enthusiastic. Virtually all the women in amateur porn share that quality—enthusiasm. They are actually enjoying themselves: the activities, the violation of taboos, the exhibitionism. Clearly, there's no coercion here.

In contrast to the typically grim, ideological anti-porn critique, our analysis of porn's attraction and value *would* predict and *can* explain why amateur porn is such a rapidly growing genre. If the keys to porn's popularity are validation of the viewer's vision of erotic abundance, female lust, and the reasonableness of erotic focus, a viewer can experience those even more intensely when this validation comes not from actors but from real people. Rather than actors *implying* that the viewer isn't alone, amateur photos and video show real people *proving* the viewer isn't alone.

So what does the viewer of amateur porn see? Everyday folks being lusty, exhibiting themselves, and participating in an erotic community. It's a community where sexuality is understood as wholesome even when it's expressed in taboo ways.

PORNOGRAPHY'S TRUTHS AS SUBVERSIVE

And why does our culture resist these truths? Because the revolutionary implications of empowering people sexually challenge the cultural status quo. Pornography does this without even portraying sex exactly as most people experience it.

Pornography is an admission that human beings feel, imagine, and do what they do. In a culture committed to both hiding and pathologizing (and therefore shaming) sex as it really is, this admission isn't polite. It's subversive.

Ultimately, pornography's truths are subversive because they claim that we can empower ourselves and create our own erotic norms. Political structures just hate when ideas or cultural products empower people. This is the recurring lesson of Copernicus, Guttenberg, Margaret Sanger, Lenny Bruce, Timothy Leary, and Martin Luther King, Jr. In the conventional fear/danger model, the genders are adversaries. Pornography shows a reconciliation of the war of the sexes, as it contains no adversaries. In most of it, everyone shares the same interests: passion, unself-consciousness, self-acceptance, pleasure, and mutuality. Porn undermines the conventional scarcity-themed sexual economy and gender hierarchy; this is one of its most radical features, and is a big reason it attracts political opposition.

The massive popularity of pornography, and its consistent themes of female lust and male-female mutuality, testify to our pain about the conventional sexual economy. Taking porn on its own terms would require society to acknowledge this pain; such a cultural challenge makes pornography subversive.

Porn is subversive because it says that sex is not dangerous.

AMERICA'S CONVERSATION ABOUT PORN: ONE HAND CLAPPING

The format of America's cultural conversation about pornography reveals a great deal.

- It focuses almost exclusively on negativity.
- It depends on misinformation and mythology.
- Critics claim they don't use the product, but claim expertise on the product's content (and its effects on users and the community).
- Almost no one will stand up for mainstream pornography.
- People who do stand up for it are perceived as immoral, anti-family, anti-child, and anti-woman.

What does this mean? Doesn't anyone notice that there is an activity done by 50 million people that practically no one will stand up and defend? And that anyone who does defend it is personally attacked? Gun ownership is controversial, but both its practitioners and critics defend their positions passionately—each actually proselytizes, hoping to convert others. Drinking alcohol is demonstrably harmful for a percentage of drinkers and for innocent bystanders; but alcohol distributors extol their product enthusiastically, no one ever suggests banning it for adults, and all but the most destructive drinkers are considered normal or even cool.

So what does the current one-sided monologue *mean?* What does it mean when one part of society discusses the behavior (and consciousness) of the other, and the voice of that other is missing?

It means that we hear only about porn's "victims." It means anti-porn activists can maintain the illusion that porn is a pathetic activity for marginalized people. This isn't healthy for our Republic's integrity.

Every anti-porn fundraising appeal, every government hearing, every op-ed piece shouts that porn is everywhere, that it's taken over, that it's a multibillion dollar industry. Then they say porn is "attempting" to be mainstream—as if it isn't already. They say porn is on the margins of our culture trying to get in and infect "normal" society—while simultaneously complaining that everything is "pornified" and that we must "reclaim" our culture.

But to say that porn is simultaneously everywhere and marginalized is a willfully distorted interpretation of the reality critics themselves describe. With 50 million viewers, half of all Internet searches, $12 billion spent annually (more than all the tickets to professional baseball, basketball, and football combined), porn is the mainstream entertainment choice of America. The fact that most people won't talk about their choice, and that non-viewers damn this choice, doesn't change the fact. Viewing porn is a central American activity.

Why don't porn consumers speak up when they hear themselves mocked, pitied, attacked, feared, dehumanized? When the fury of enraged neighbors is whipped up by the bully pulpits of the ignorant and authoritarian, and supported by the legal machinery of city and state—all arrayed against their choice of entertainment, which they experience as harmless?

It's because people who consume porn have learned to hide it. You mention it to your neighbor, and maybe your kids can't play there anymore. Your neighbor mentions it to his poker buddy, and maybe you lose a customer, or a promotion. If you suggest it to your wife and she watches Maury, Tyra, Nancy, Anderson, Geraldo, Katie, or Dr. Phil—or any show on the Christian Broadcasting Network or Trinity Broadcasting Network—you may regret it for the rest of your life.

Religious training has instilled a tremendous shame in many porn consumers. That doesn't stop them from using it (guilt can actually drive usage),[30] only from feeling comfortable about it—and feeling they have a legitimate right to it.

The unending, escalating propaganda about porn leading to violence and child endangerment means that defending the right to use porn (say, in a letter to the editor about a local vigilante group) invites the wrath of a righteous mob that no sane person wants. And with the successful demonization of "pornographers," no one wants to be associated with those sub-humans.

Americans have had so many rights of expression, economic choice, and privacy for so long, that most have trouble envisioning their world without them. For people who enjoy a little porn once a week, it's hard to imagine our country's constitutional structure turning on such a seemingly trivial thing. The righteous anger of the Right, enthroned in federal and state government, clearly sees what the average porn consumer still doesn't—the profound connection between the personal and the political.

DEFENDING DEMOCRACY

Finally, we have to say that there's more at stake in the war on porn than the right to look at a picture of a friendly lady's nipples. It just so happens that sexuality/pornography is the vehicle of the moment in the eternal tug-of-war about the nature and meaning of the American system. At various times, that vehicle has been race (separate-but-equal; Japanese internment camps); age (child labor law, mandatory education); and private property rights (eminent domain, anti-discrimination law). Similarly, religion is another contemporary vehicle in this tug-of-war (stem-cell research, right to die, school vouchers, school prayer, Christmas displays on public property).

Pornography might not be the battlefield on which you or I would choose to defend secular pluralism, free expression, and science-based (as opposed to emotion-based) public policy. But as this is the battlefield that has been chosen for us, we must respond with energy and vision, neither apologizing nor acquiescing to manipulative descriptions of what porn is, who porn consumers are, or what the fight over porn is about.

The increasingly aggressive and confident attacks on porn are based on the following assumptions:

- The right to look at porn is constitutionally trivial.
- The social benefits from limiting/banning porn are huge.
- The social and personal costs of limiting/banning porn are virtually zero.
- Limiting/banning porn doesn't harm the American system.

Resisting the War on Sex requires articulating these assumptions, discussing their importance to all Americans, and then challenging every single one. Those who want to eliminate porn justify their extreme proposals by saying that the stakes are too high for halfway measures or fey concerns about free expression. They're absolutely right—the stakes are very, very high.

Chapter Thirteen

EXTREME RELIGION AND PUBLIC POLICY

I am pro-life. So are you.
So was Saddam Hussein. And Hitler.
So were Lincoln and the guy who killed him.
And John Lennon and the guy who killed him.
Every mass murderer is pro-life.
The question is—which life, or lives, does a person mean by "pro-life"?

Who gets to decide? Why? The American system is not allowed to assume that one person's ideas about "life" are more legitimate than anyone else's, even if that person is "religious." The idea that government policy should reflect any religious belief is rejected by our Constitution.

Our system creates a civic paradox that some find uncomfortable:

- The government is forbidden to dictate what you believe, so . . .
  You're allowed to believe anything you want, so . . .
- You can join with your fellow believers and influence public policy,
  but . . .
- Only to the extent that it doesn't intrude on the expression of others'
  beliefs—or limit the expression of their Constitutional rights.

That's the genius of America, the feature that has enabled our country to prosper while functioning as a multicultural melting pot: Give everyone the same chance, and don't let officials or groups dictate what citizens believe in private. This allows everyone to have dignity and personal power, no matter how poor they are or how idiosyncratic their beliefs. This is exactly what was missing from multicultural societies that imploded in the last 20 years, from Yugoslavia to Iraq.

When Iran issued its infamous 1990 fatwa against Salman Rushdie, many in the West were indignant about a political regime passing a death sentence on someone simply for articulating a "blasphemous" thought.[1]

Western Europe is now struggling with the early breakdown of their social contract of pluralism and tolerance. The 2004 assassination of Dutch film-maker Theo van Gogh for criticizing Islam's treatment of women was a shocking challenge to the principle that people with contradictory religious ideas can coexist in civil society. Early in 2006, Denmark grappled with its Islamic community's reaction to newspaper cartoons they said insulted the Prophet Muhammad. Local Muslims said they were "mentally tortured" by the images, and wanted the public expression of certain ideas forbidden. The newspaper, of course, was well within the West's normal rights of free expression, but the artist received death threats. In subsequent months, over a million Muslims in dozens of countries marched in protest, almost always resulting in violence and, to date, hundreds of deaths.[2]

Islamic preachers throughout the world are now explicitly calling for the destruction of the Western political system. They do not want non-Muslims to have even the limited rights of self-expression that Muslims do. In February 2006, Sheikh Hassan Nasrallah told hundreds of thousands of Shia followers in Beirut that "We want the European parliament to draft laws that ban newspapers from insulting the Prophet."[3] The stark irony that it is precisely in the West that Muslims may express their ideas more fully than in any Muslim country on earth, of course, completely escapes these religious zealots.

It seems clear that more assassinations, accompanied by increasing numbers of people inhibiting what they say, write, and draw will surely follow. *While pluralism makes room for religious fundamentalism, religious fundamentalism wishes to destroy pluralism.* This asymmetry is an enormous political advantage for religious fundamentalism.

Similarly, zealous American Christians believe they are called upon to shape the public policy of the country in which they live. They believe that everyone should follow the word of the Christian god, even those who don't believe in that god, or who interpret that god's word differently. They might be called the Christian-American Taliban. They have murdered physicians and medical staff, and seriously wounded innocent bystanders. Like the white racists who firebombed churches in the South, they have firebombed medical clinics providing legal services they want criminalized.

The ferocity, the lying, the emotional and physical violence in which these people are willing to engage make it clear that they are involved in a fundamentally different struggle than the daily civic strife of healthy democracy. Their behavior sounds like news reports from Pakistan, not the United States. Indeed, political animosity in America goes all the way back to Founders such as Thomas Jefferson, John Adams, and Thomas Paine, who passionately and quite publicly hated their rivals' positions. But they all agreed on how to stay engaged in a common process during conflict, and sought to create a country that guaranteed that same American dream for their countrymen. They didn't bomb each other's homes or churches.

American Christianity is extremely heterogeneous. Many Christians celebrate pluralism and the reality of different beliefs—including non-belief—in their communities and the world. But today's religious zealots, like James Dobson, Michele Bachmann, Gary Bauer, Glenn Beck, Brent Bozell, Pat Robertson, Penny Nance, and Rick Santorum, do not agree with their opponents on the rules of the game. They say they do not want to govern a pluralistic, secular democracy; they want to govern a country whose goals are fundamentally different than America's have ever been, whose citizens have fundamentally different rights than we have today.

They see a powerful connection between non-believers' sexuality and their own. They believe their world is being polluted by the sexuality of non-believers. Conceptualizing their world as being vulnerable to others' sexual sin almost inevitably leads to warring on the sexuality of non-believers in order to take care of themselves.

And most importantly, they see this battle as far bigger than mere earthly issues of pluralism, democracy, and individual rights. And so legal, cultural, social, even spiritual appeals to traditional American pluralism can't succeed, because they don't live in a world in which they can be safe if others are not like them. And so Randall Terry will go to jail 40 times, James Kopp will murder physicians who happen to perform abortions, and other religious terrorists—individually, in groups, or as elected officials—will pursue an America exactly as theocratic (no more, no less) as Iran.

Americans can no longer count on elected officials to uphold the single most important principle of American government and society—that everyone has the right to their own opinion, and has the right to live their own non-violent life as they please. This war is no metaphor. The struggle is tangible, and sexual expression is a key battlefield on which the war for the American covenant is being fought.

If these people did not claim to be devoutly religious—if, say, they were inspired by alcoholism, or visions of King Tut, or a desire to return the Louisiana Purchase to France—their demands would receive little serious consideration (and wouldn't be tax-exempt). But because they say their program is driven by religious considerations, they get a seat at America's public policy table. And so their bizarre demand that, for example, every American be prevented from using contraceptives or having abortions is taken seriously, included as a legitimate voice in public debate—because they claim this is the demand of their god. Even the one million people promoting citizenship and civil rights for fertilized eggs ("protecting the pre-born," they call it) are taken seriously—because they claim their idea is motivated by religion rather than by schizophrenia or comedy.[4]

The very idea that sexuality is a religious issue, that public policy about sexuality requires the input of religious leaders, that religious leaders have special expertise about sexuality and public policy (because it involves what they call morality), is just an opinion—primarily the opinion of religious believers. The fact that so many people now accept the pragmatic inevitability of this linkage is itself a profound anti-sex victory in the War on Sex. (Once again validating the peculiar idea that "morality" is about limiting sexual expression.)

Given the high visibility and political influence afforded religious leaders today, which voices will be heard in the public square? For three decades, it has increasingly been the least tolerant, most anti-sex figures. If moderate or sex-positive religious leaders and laypeople cannot recapture their organizations from radicals who threaten our democracy, secular, pluralistically minded people will have to protect our democracy from them. This terrifying struggle is giving all American religion a bad name. The mass media is complicit in this, giving religious radicals far more exposure than moderates because their extreme, divisive opinions make for dramatic, conflict-oriented shows and stories.

In *Planned Parenthood v. Casey* (1992), the Supreme Court declared it is up to each individual to determine "the concept of existence, of meaning, of the universe, and of the mystery of human life."[5] This summarizes what makes America different from Saudi Arabia, North Korea, and other totalitarian societies. Every American is expected to agree to tolerate his neighbors' wacky ideas about the meaning of life in exchange for tolerance of his own ideas. The lack of this single idea led to hundreds of years of brutal religious warfare in Western Europe.

In contrast, Pope John Paul II warned against this very "alliance between democracy and ethical relativism." *Christianity Today* says, "This means that when truth itself is democratized—when truth is no more than the will of each individual or a majority of individuals—democracy is deprived of the claim to truth and stands naked to its enemies."[6]

By "truth," they and the Pope mean religious belief. By "truth," the Supreme Court means scientific truth—that is, facts. This truth is not up for referendum. Gravity exists whether people believe in it or not. Racism and sexism have real, measurable consequences. Similarly, belief is not up for referendum. People believe what they believe, no matter how little grounded in fact or possibility. Truth is eternal, and belief is eternal. But they

Breaking the Law to Protect God

The following has been summarized from Joshua Green's fine article in the *Atlantic*, which appeared in October 2005.

Soon after taking office as Chief Justice of the Alabama Supreme Court in 2001, Roy Moore caused a national uproar by commissioning and installing a granite monument of the Ten Commandments in the state Supreme Court building and refusing to remove it. In the summer of 2003, "Roy's Rock" was the focus of intense debate about the government's proper relationship to religion. When Moore defied a federal court order to remove the monument, supporters from across the country descended on Montgomery, living on the steps of the Supreme Court building, and praying, singing, threatening, blowing ram's horns—all to protect God from the government's latest assault. After the conflict went to the U.S. Supreme Court, Moore was removed from office for disobeying the federal court order.

Here's the climax of Attorney General Bill Pryor's 2003 cross-examination of Alabama Chief Justice Roy Moore, on trial for disregarding a federal court order preventing him from displaying a 5,000-pound religious sculpture of the Ten Commandments in his courthouse:

Pryor: And your understanding is that the federal court ordered that you could not acknowledge God; isn't that right?

Moore: Yes.

Pryor: And if you resume your duties as Chief Justice after this proceeding, you will continue to acknowledge God as you have testified that you would today?

Moore: That's right.

Pryor: No matter what any other official says?

Moore: Absolutely. Let me clarify that. Without an acknowledgment of God, I cannot do my duties. I must acknowledge God . . .

Pryor: If you do resume your duties as Chief Justice, you will continue to do that without regard to what any other official says. Isn't that right?

Moore: . . . I think you must.[a]

[a]Joshua Green, "Roy and His Rock," *Atlantic Online*, October 2005, http://www.theatlantic.com/doc/200510/roy-moores-ten-commandments.

are not the same thing. When belief is elevated above truth, when religion and "morality" are taken as some ultimate, factual measure for law, democracy is deprived of the claim to truth and does stand naked to its enemies. We all hate that this enslaves a hundred million people in Iran and its neighbors. We must prevent it from taking over here as well.[7]

BELIEF VERSUS ACTION

No matter how misplaced, many of the battles to control and limit Americans' sexual expression have a heartfelt component. In addition to (ill-informed) practical concerns ("porn causes rape," "sex on TV hurts kids," "contraception causes sterility"), people often invoke "moral" considerations (teens shouldn't be sexual, pornography enables infidelity). These "moral" concerns are particularly common in the battle over reproductive rights/abortion.

Abortion can be located in morality (both the autonomy of the woman and the value of fetal life), complete subjectivity (when does life begin), a tiny bit of science (ditto), and some (mostly recent) religious doctrine. Thus, those opposing abortion can sound like they're on solid ground—that at the very least, their argument is as legitimate as any other. But it's a familiar, multifaceted program—attempting to control everyone's sexuality, saying anything necessary to justify it, even referring to an alleged "culture of life" (which is ad hoc nonsense, given their other public policy positions).

Some people claim a religious doctrinaire approach to oppose abortion and contraception. History shows that this argument is an artifact of political, very human decision-making. No less than St. Augustine (fifth century), Pope Innocent (thirteenth century), and St. Thomas Aquinas (thirteenth century) believed abortion in the first trimester was at times acceptable. Pope Sixtus (sixteenth century) said abortion at any stage was murder and should be punishable by death; only three years later, Pope Gregory reversed this, accepting abortion through 16½ weeks of pregnancy. So today's Christian who screams that all abortion is murder would be condemning several cherished saints and popes.

In 1869, Pope Pius IX once again reversed the Catholic Church's tolerant stance on abortion, where it has remained for 137 years—just a mere coffee break in the 20 centuries of Church time.

The construct of Limbo was adopted almost a thousand years ago as the destination of unbaptized infants' souls; Pope Benedict recently started eliminating it, wanting it replaced by a more "compassionate" doctrine.[8]

No American is prevented from believing what he or she wants about abortion or Limbo. But when the Church changes its position on abortion or Limbo again in a decade, a century, or a millennium, presumably the rights it will support for non-believers will change again. Will believers then apologize for how they have forced, or tried to force, non-believers to live?

YEARNING FOR THE SIMPLE, YEARNING FOR THE DIVINE

Complex times such as ours demand a great deal of self-direction and confidence from individuals. The wish for a simple morality to help one through complex times is understandable. Some people also yearn to connect with the Divine, and, of course, that's a key promise of religious observance. Americans who want this, though, typically want it now, not after a lifetime of meditation and prayer. So for those who want to connect with the Divine now, acquiring ritual purity has far more appeal than painstakingly developing actual ("moral") purity. For many people, that's what religion is for: to tell them what they can do to have certifiable contact with the Divine.

Many Christian spiritual leaders have said that the key is doing good works. Jesus himself proposed that getting to heaven involved, more than anything else, helping others in tangible ways (see Matthew 25). But for some Christian fundamentalists, the modern route to heaven isn't so much what you *do*, it's what you *believe*—which is a lot easier. It can be done with virtually no sacrifice of position or comfort or time.

So for many fundamentalist Christians these days, the way to experience the Divine is to believe. And how do you show that you really believe? By attempting to force others to act the way you think is right. Wanting other people to forego behavior you think is immoral is a very low-cost way to feel religiously intact. Write a check, vote for an anti-choice candidate, go to church and commune with those who also believe. No sacrifice—just force others to sacrifice.

In some Christian sects, being against unauthorized sex is a certifiable way to contact the Divine. Conceptualizing "unauthorized sex," of course, is the first step. Attacking sex is a way to live in the modern world and feel spiritual, without foregoing the comforts of technology or material goods.

The Abrahamic religions have problematized the body. Early influential Christian philosophers, such as Tertullian and Anicius Boethius, called woman "a temple built over a sewer."[9] At various times, Judaism has been obsessed with seminal emissions and menstrual impurity. Islam's fixation on covering women's bodies is well documented.

Believers, therefore, have to "solve" this "problem." Seeing sex as the representative of the body calls for a philosophical policy about it, and seeing sexuality in a highly limited way makes this project much easier. Conceptualizing sexuality as impure then simply presents the religious community the task of purifying it. That means limiting those who would be pure to two choices: authorized sex or no sex.

With the two most revered figures in Christian history (Jesus and the Virgin Mary) both considered celibate (and she celebrated for that far beyond other qualities such as compassion or wisdom—it's her name!), there's a limit to how much believers can embrace sexuality and still feel spiritual. Eschewing eroticism (however that is intellectually justified) is a far more internally coherent solution to this Christian dilemma. And so any rationalizations that conceptualize and then condemn "uncontrolled" or "unspiritual" sex are very convenient.

In fact, today's fundamentalist Christians are often *pietistic*; they observe or profess *beyond* what's required, as a way of making a statement about themselves to themselves. Piety reinforces one's self-identification as spiritual. It is always symbolic at its core, which makes it easier to profess than to actually live Jesus's project of empowering the powerless. Jesus never said, "Fighting abortion is more important than feeding the poor." But it is easier, cleaner, more exciting, and it doesn't upset the neighborhood. Similarly, Jesus never said, "Since your time is limited, and you can't rescue everyone, care about the unborn more than the born. Way more."

But somehow, that's what millions of Christians are choosing to rescue—the unborn, rather than the born—and choosing to adopt—frozen embryos instead of warm foster children. How are they choosing their projects? Apparently, to maximize their political impact. Not coincidentally, they keep selecting projects that limit others' sexual choices. Their War on Sex around reproduction helps them feel holy, although it doesn't help (and demonstrably harms) the disadvantaged already living.

It isn't that the Right has no heart, it's that it applies its heart to causes that pay off in controlling sexuality. So it claims it cares for "degraded" porn actresses, "vulnerable" prostitutes, and heartbroken teenagers. It doesn't show the same concern for poor women who need day care, immigrant women who need English classes, or single women who need contraception to avoid pregnancies that will damage or destroy their families.

Many leaders of the Religious Right explicitly say their goal is installing a moral, Christ-centered government in the United States. That is, they want a government that will abandon America's 236-year-long tradition of pluralism. That is, they want to change the most fundamental rules of America. And if 51 percent of America votes for this, or if 99 percent of America votes for this, it will still be wrong. It certainly won't be "traditionally" American.

GOVERNMENTAL COLLUSION

America's religiously themed anti-sex program couldn't succeed without active, enthusiastic government action. So why have America's federal and state governments fallen in with these repressive elements?

There are presumably a variety of reasons, but they are primarily the twin evils of politics—money and power, along with something rarely found in

American government—personal belief. And the impact of the irrational belief is enhanced because of the piety factor described above.

Former President George W. Bush described himself as ardently "pro-life" and has said he believes the laws of America should reflect his religious beliefs as much as possible. In 2002, he declared January 18 the first annual Sanctity of Life Day, describing America's "essential moral duties, including . . . caring for children born and unborn." And when he signed a 2004 bill recognizing that fetuses have rights separate from the mothers carrying them, he said, "We reaffirm that the United States of America is building a culture of life."[10]

Thousands of other American politicians explicitly say they are attempting to inject Christian values into American governance. And former Alabama Chief Justice Roy Moore says God is the basis of American government—his vision amounting, according to the *Atlantic*, to "a theocracy." "Let every soul be subject unto the higher powers," says Moore. "Separation of church and state does not mean separation of God and government! We must return God to our public life and restore the moral foundation of our law."[11]

In 2000, presidential candidate Pat Buchanan said that RU-486 is an abomination to God, and therefore, if elected, "I would use all the power of my office, including FDA appointments, to prevent RU-486 from being put on the market." Note the logic: Buchanan's decision that *his* god disapproves of RU-486 is the reason that all Americans, including those who don't believe that Buchanan's god exists, should be denied access to this medication. How different is this from saying that since Elvis would disapprove, no one should have access to the drug?

This idealism is horribly misguided, a fundamental misunderstanding of the American system. But it is idealism nevertheless. Unfortunately, that means that not even a high-quality civics lesson would be enough to change such attitudes about the role of belief in democratic government. There is no difference between President Bush and Judge Moore saying, "The law must conform to my religious beliefs" and Ayatollah Khamenei and President Ahmadinejad saying, "The law must conform to my religious beliefs."

Money and power are the more sinister reasons that politicians are attempting to destroy Americans' reproductive rights—and their influence, of course, is everywhere. Churches and religious organizations are giving more money to political candidates and officials than ever before. And in return, the government is giving churches and religious groups more money than ever before.

President Bush's 2001 "faith-based initiative" (which President Obama *expanded*) was an honest declaration of his intention to do so, and he was extremely effective. Under this plan, tens of millions of federal tax dollars were distributed to religious (i.e., Christian) ministries to provide social services that were historically provided by government agencies or secular

Religious Pluralism

Fortunately, not all religious believers are intent on controlling others' behavior, whether through forced conversions, or by changing the laws to criminalize that which they consider sinful and requiring that which their god demands.

There has always been a tolerant side to the American religious tradition, expressed variously by Quakers, the civil rights movement, social justice theology, and the 1960s/1970s anti-war movement. Now that sexuality is the focus of so much hostile and dangerous religious input into public policy, America desperately needs that religious tolerance.

And so, the Religious Institute on Sexual Morality, Justice, and Healing was founded in 2001. Now directed by Reverend Debra Haffner, it advocates for sexual health, education, and justice in faith communities and society. It supports religious leaders and congregations in creating sexually healthy faith communities.

The Institute has published an historical declaration, now endorsed by more than 2,500 religious leaders from dozens of traditions. As a reminder of how religion and sexual health can passionately coexist, and as a way of honoring the Institute's life-affirming work in a sexually hostile world, the declaration is reproduced here in full. Readers are encouraged to find out more at http://www.religiousinstitute.org.

Religious Declaration on Sexual Morality, Justice, and Healing

Sexuality is God's life-giving and life-fulfilling gift. We come from diverse religious communities to recognize sexuality as central to our humanity and as integral to our spirituality. We are speaking out against the pain, brokenness, oppression, and loss of meaning that many experience about their sexuality.

Our faith traditions celebrate the goodness of creation, including our bodies and our sexuality. We sin when this sacred gift is abused or exploited. However, the great promise of our traditions is love, healing, and restored relationships.

Our culture needs a sexual ethic focused on personal relationships and social justice rather than particular sexual acts. All persons have the right and responsibility to lead sexual lives that express love, justice, mutuality, commitment, consent, and pleasure. Grounded in respect for the body and for the vulnerability that intimacy brings, this ethic fosters physical, emotional, and spiritual health. It accepts no double standards and applies to all persons, without regard to sex, gender, color, age, bodily condition, marital status, or sexual orientation.

God hears the cries of those who suffer from the failure of religious communities to address sexuality. We are called today to see, hear, and respond to the suffering caused by violence against women and sexual minorities, the HIV pandemic, unsustainable population growth and over-consumption, and the commercial exploitation of sexuality.

Faith communities must therefore be truth-seeking, courageous, and just. We call for:

- Theological reflection that integrates the wisdom of excluded, often silenced peoples, and insights about sexuality from medicine, social science, the arts and humanities.
- Full inclusion of women and sexual minorities in congregational life, including their ordination and the blessing of same sex unions.
- Sexuality counseling and education throughout the lifespan from trained religious leaders.
- Support for those who challenge sexual oppression and who work for justice within their congregations and denomination.

Faith communities must also advocate for sexual and spiritual wholeness in society. We call for:

- Lifelong, age appropriate sexuality education in schools, seminaries, and community settings.
- A faith-based commitment to sexual and reproductive rights, including access to voluntary contraception, abortion, and HIV/STD prevention and treatment.
- Religious leadership in movements to end sexual and social injustice.

God rejoices when we celebrate our sexuality with holiness and integrity. We, the undersigned, invite our colleagues and faith communities to join us in promoting sexual morality, justice, and healing.

grantees, including health care "counseling," abstinence education, afterschool programs, job training, drug treatment, prison rehabilitation, and pregnancy "counseling."

For example, Herb Lusk is a Philadelphia preacher with a long history of partisan activity on behalf of Republicans. In 2006, his Greater Exodus Baptist Church hosted a nationally broadcast rally to support the confirmation of

Supreme Court nominee Samuel Alito. Sponsored by the Family Research Council, speakers included Jerry Falwell, Tony Perkins, James Dobson, and Senator Rick Santorum (who was facing a tight reelection campaign).[12]

Reverend Lusk was awarded $1.4 million of taxpayers' money in faith-based grants by the Bush administration—and despite his work's obviously partisan nature, he can administer the funds through tax-exempt organizations. Is his passion for Alito or for money and power? According to the *New York Times*, Lusk said, "I don't know enough about him to actually think he's the right man to do the job."[13]

Another personal cause of President Bush was so-called embryo adoption. At a 2005 press conference on stem cell research, he introduced an (now federally funded) agency, Nightlight Christian Adoption. He spoke of the value of human life, saying that there is no such thing as a "spare embryo." Twenty-one children born from adopted embryos ("snowflake children") were paraded on stage to, as the agency director put it, "put a face to these embryos under discussion."[14]

This pattern is repeated in abstinence programs, crisis pregnancy centers, and other tax-exempt religious institutions across America—state and federal officials funnel money to local and national groups, which support these officials and elect others. These groups now brazenly boast of their influence in destroying Americans' reproductive rights: Concerned Women for America, for example, listed thwarting over-the-counter sales of the morning-after pill as one of its 2005 accomplishments.[15]

CHALLENGING AMERICA'S COVENANT

The U.S. Constitution guarantees each of us the freedom to practice any religion. This freedom does not extend to challenging the fundamental principle of the United States, that your freedom ends where my nose (or uterus) begins. Regardless of the majority's wishes, fundamental principles like these can never be put up for referendum.

Somehow, those against the public's access to contraceptive technology have put this access up for referendum. Each side continues scrambling for adherents. This means that those opposed to the unlimited availability of contraceptives have already won a crucial victory in the War on Sex. Wouldn't we say the same thing if slavery were put up for a vote? Regardless of who won such a vote, the forces of freedom and democracy would have lost.

Chapter Fourteen

BATTLEGROUND: SEXUAL PRIVACY AND SEXUAL MINORITIES—CIVIL RIGHTS OR IMMORAL PRIVILEGES?

It's hard to believe, but in America today, who you make love with, and how, actually determines what your rights are—both in and out of your bedroom.

Yes, the government uses your sexual preferences and orientation to help decide if you should get custody of your kids, get a security clearance at your job, or be allowed to practice your sexual hobby in private. And if the government doesn't approve of your sexual interests, you won't be allowed to buy the toys you want, gather with strangers to have sex, or kiss your partner in public. Your sexual preferences even help determine whether you get fully competent services from a physician, attorney, or therapist.

Up until late 2011, your sexual orientation determined whether you'd be welcome to serve in the U.S. military, regardless of your qualifications to protect the country. In 2002, for example, just a year after 9/11, the Army discharged nine linguists, including six fluent in Arabic, for being gay.[1]

For decades, a variety of Christian groups have demanded that America pursue this prejudice more energetically and punitively. They were behind the nineteenth-century Comstock ban on selling or mailing contraceptives, the 1930s Hays code that censored Hollywood films, and J. Edgar Hoover's post-war FBI drive to identify and punish homosexuals in the government and public life. You can see it in the thousand dollars the First Baptist Church in Huntingburg, Indiana, donated to Spencer County to help county commissioners get rid of the local Love Boutique. Separation of (tax-exempt) church and state, anyone?[2]

The central question, almost beyond belief in a modern country, is: Do all Americans have to have sex the same way in order to claim their fair share of the American dream, or of American justice? To people obsessed with "normal" sex, the answer is yes.

You may think this has nothing to do with you. "I'm not gay and I'm not kinky," you might say. "I'm sympathetic to people who get busted for being either one, but that's just the way it is. And it's not my problem."

Wrong.

Because once the government can pathologize any kind of sex, it can pathologize any kind of sex—even yours.

And although your sexual interests may currently be perfectly legal (the very idea that private sex has to be declared "legal" is itself chilling), what if you experiment with something new and like it? Or you get involved with a new partner who likes something you never thought about? Or some local group decides that what you now enjoy is dangerous for the community? You could find yourself a sexual fugitive faster than you think. Because like all wars do, the War on Sex is creating refugees everywhere.

Today, some 30 million tax-paying, otherwise law-abiding Americans are in danger—not because they hurt others or others' property, but because they enjoy certain kinds of sex in private. Whether they're gay, or into S/M, or they swing with their spouse, they have fewer rights than others do. Despite their enormous numbers, they live as part of a sexual minority.

The creation of sexual minorities—groups who are disenfranchised or in danger because their sexual interests are disapproved of—is dangerous not just for people in those groups. It's also dangerous for those who are not part of a sexual minority.

The sex under attack doesn't have to be extreme sex, doesn't have to hurt anyone, doesn't even have to generate any complaints. It can be as innocuous as riding the glass elevator at the Hyatt Regency without panties. Or your professor overhearing your girlfriend talk about the rough sex you both like. That's why you should care.

To give you a bird's-eye view, laws that were recently passed by America's state or local governments have punished citizens who:

- Played an X-rated videotape in a moving car
- Paid to get an erotic spanking at a strip club
- Had rough sex with a consenting adult
- Went to a private swing club and watched his wife give a friend a blow job
- Sold sex toys at a party of adults who invited her

And don't forget the four-star general who lost his job for having sex with a civilian who wasn't his wife—even though they're in the middle of an amicable divorce and neither woman complained.[3]

The prevailing Big Lie is that "giving" sexual minorities civil rights somehow undermines the rights of everyone else—and, of course, sends the "wrong message" (of tolerance, how ugly). We should consider the other side—how, ironically, depriving sexual minorities of their civil rights undermines the freedom of all Americans.

WHY PUBLIC-IZE SEXUALITY? (PRONOUNCED "PUBLIC EYES")

Remember, "sexuality" is much more than intercourse or genital stimulation.

So is private sex in America, um, private?

It depends on whom you ask.

Those who fear sex conceptualize all sex as public. They have a well-worn list of ways that private, consensual, adult sexual behavior supposedly affects the community, and is therefore not really private. If your private sexual behavior doesn't meet their criteria for "normal," they believe that it:

- Hurts children (always the number one reason for restricting sexual rights)
- Undermines other people's conventional marriages
- Encourages "sex addiction" (to vibrators, S/M, or whatever individuals do)
- Exploits women (always a great reason for restricting any sexual rights)
- Disrespects the God-fearing community
- Encourages masturbation (which is presumed to be a bad thing)

People who believe this think your sexuality is their business. Many of them want to use the law to establish moral norms and express social disapproval. This was Justice Antonin Scalia's reason that the Supreme Court should keep anal sex illegal when he dissented in *Lawrence v. Texas* in 2003. As Professor Strossen noted in this book's foreword, Justice Scalia warned that state laws against bigamy, same-sex marriage, adult incest, prostitution, masturbation, adultery, fornication, bestiality, and obscenity would be vulnerable if Texas's ban on sodomy was overturned. With a few exceptions,[4] that hasn't happened.

And there's a deeper, more personal concern at work, which may not even be conscious. Many people who fear sex in general learn, in childhood, to fear their own sexuality. More than almost any other Western country, America is filled with family, religious, and community environments that teach children that their sexuality is bad. Growing up, they project this internalized eroto-phobia outward, onto others. The simple unconscious logic is, "If my sexuality is dangerous, so is my neighbor's."

For people caught in such a bind, the easiest way to reduce anxiety about their own sexuality is to repress others'—that is, *yours*. They then rationalize their anxiety-reduction strategy of controlling your sexuality: "I owe it to my family/community/God." Your private sexuality then becomes everybody's business.

Thus, public-izing private sexuality is an effective way of addressing one's fear of others' sexuality. This explains the desire for censorship, even of one-self—eliminating sexual opportunities for others, because one's own self can't be trusted.

A lot of public policy is unconsciously formulated and consciously presented as a response to public need, when it's really a response to personal need. This explains why some people are so obsessed with regulating others' sexual behavior and decision-making. And it's absolutely predictable that they would see sex everywhere, providing a never-ending source of energy to repress it.

Since these frightened people conceptualize all sex as public, they feel enti-tled to demand that the government control everyone's sexual behavior. That was the justification for criminalizing sex between people of different races, contraception for single people, and anal sex. And why it's still illegal in much of America to lie on a beach nude even when no one's complaining, or to gather behind the closed doors of a private club and have sex with strangers.

Many of these frightened people also say they are called by their religion to set the rules for everyone's sexual expression, regardless of the rights our sec-ular government ensures each of us. And they think that because they credit their impulses to religion rather than to narcissism, paranoia, erotophobia, or their own early trauma, they actually have the right to do so. Whether they phrase this gently ("We want everyone to enjoy the advantages of our way of life") or harshly ("We must prevent others from living differently from us"), their intention is the same.

In reality, religious conservatives are just a powerful, radical pressure group that threatens American pluralism and tolerance. Why should swing club owners be considered just a self-interested lobby, while a group trying to eliminate a town's swing clubs is considered the "community voice" or "com-munity activists"? Similarly, why are those who aren't prejudiced against gays adopting kids considered "the gay lobby," while those who oppose it are considered "the public" or "the voice of America's families"?

The idea that "all sex ultimately accrues to the community" must be met with the psychological and political truth that "the *results* of public-izing all sex accrues to the community." When sexual expression is repressed, when individuals' rights are routinely violated and they are made to feel guilty, everyone suffers. Consciously or not, most people struggle with "normality anxiety."[5] The community must cope with the anger, acting out (sexual and nonsexual), secrecy, and even addictions provoked by the resulting guilt and restrictions. Society can't repress something as fundamental as sexual orientation or sexual expression without paying a price in reduced mental health and community safety.

SEX, CLEAN AND DIRTY

With sex in America firmly public-ized, how are "clean" and "dirty" sex to be differentiated? That's the principal conceit behind criminalizing certain sexual expression. It's commonplace to note that non-reproductive sex is often considered dirty, but the issue goes beyond that. Attached to reproduction or not, anti-sex people feel that passion is dirty, lust is dirty, pleasure itself is suspect, even within the context of monogamous, heterosexual intercourse. This is even more true for other erotic configurations. Sexual intensity, then, is the enemy, and virtually anything done to increase the intensity of sexual arousal or experience is problematic. For those afraid of sex, in fact, that's the definition of kinky: anything that attempts to heighten the intensity of so-called normal sex. As recently as 50 years ago, many Americans considered oral sex kinky, done only by prostitutes and other taboo subcultures.[6] Similarly, anal sex is considered rare—except by the tens of millions of people who do it.

Sexual conservatives perceive multiple layers of clean/dirty sex. Some relationships can't be clean, so it doesn't matter what you do within them (e.g., a same-gender couple). Other relationships are clean, but the activities in them can be dirty (e.g., a monogamous wife playing the "oops I forgot my panties game" at a gas station). Some relationships and activities are clean—unless you're too lusty, which tarnishes the activity (e.g., monogamous intercourse in which the wife asks the husband to ejaculate on her face).

The public-izing of sex attempts to mobilize communities to protect the American hearth, to contain the power of sexuality. The anti-sex community fears this power can spread from one home to another like a contagion. Like heresy did. Like the 1960s did. Like feminism did. That's one reason they're so committed to maintaining the myth of kids' sexual innocence—kids are seen as the generational firewall that helps contain the contagion.

In reality, sexuality encompasses a broad range of our self: what we think and feel, do with our bodies, fantasize; how we choose partners, and how we express ourselves. More pragmatically, it involves what we wear, contraceptive choices, role-playing, toys, and more. Public-izing our sexuality attempts to limit or eliminate a broad swath of these options, which is a lot of our human heritage to lose. And Americans are not safe from further losses: As you read this, churches, morality groups, legislators, and prosecutors are busy narrowing your sexual choices even more.

Americans deserve to reclaim the intrinsic privacy of private sex. Fulfilling the American promise demands it. To do so, we need to reestablish the comprehensive concept of private sex. Outside of sex, this principle is already established throughout our culture: Personal activity is considered private unless it involves coercion, fraud, or the forced, disruptive participation of the public. Playing soccer during rush hour in the center of Times Square is, rightly, prohibited. Making love there should be, too—for exactly the same reason, no more, no less. The sex part is irrelevant.

But "There is no fixed consensus on privacy and sexuality, in spite of the fact that most people feel their bodies are private," says Kinsey Institute Executive Director, Dr. Julia Heiman.[7]

Anti-sex forces have found many ways to create a gray zone between private and public sexual expression. The War on Sex pursues that gray zone with legal, economic, and political pressure. Zoning laws, morality crusades, powerful but meaningless anecdotes, and undocumented claims of secondary effects transform private activity into gray zone activity, and gray zone activity into public activity. And so Phoenix, Arizona, was able to close private swingers' clubs by declaring them places offering "live public sex acts," and an Arkansas strip club has been forced to stop offering erotic "birthday spankings" because "people can get hurt." Alabama continues to criminalize sex toys, a policy supported by federal courts.

WHO'S ALLOWED TO PRACTICE SEX UNRESTRICTED?

Throughout history, legal or religious codes have restricted various people in expressing their sexuality: the unmarried, elderly, adolescent, mentally ill, physically handicapped, terminally ill, warriors in training, menstruating women. And, in many cultures, anyone having sex with someone of the same gender.

In most modern societies, those restrictions are either gone or facing challenges. In their place, however, Americans now face other restrictions. They're based on the discomfort and superstitions of those who legislate, and the vocal minority that alternately critiques and supports them. Whether it's a zoning board, city council, district attorney, family mediator, or police chief, the story is almost always the same: Adults shouldn't be allowed to do just any sexual thing they want, even when everyone involved consents and no one complains. Certain activities, relationships, and equipment are judged both bad for participants, and bad for the community.

Or to put it more honestly, "That stuff seems weird and it scares me," or "That stuff seems exotic and exciting and it scares me," or "If that's allowed, then other stuff that's even scarier might be allowed, and it scares me."

As New York City prosecutor (Special Victims Unit) Linda Fairstein said in 2001 when describing why she was prosecuting S/M activity that she knew was consensual, she doesn't believe that "one human being should be allowed to do that to another, even if it is consensual."[8] And as Robert Peters, President of Morality in Media says, "Conclusive scientific data is not necessary" when restricting sexual activity.[9] A bunch of people being scared or disgusted is apparently all that is. It works in Iran, it works for the Taliban, so I guess there's no reason it can't work here.

There's a word that accurately describes this policy: "discrimination." Discrimination against those who enjoy inflaming their own passion (lustism?) and against those who enjoy sexual activity of which others disapprove (kinkophobia?). When people are denied rights simply because society disapproves of who they are or what they do, it's called discrimination. Kinkophobia and lustism are like racism and sexism. Remember when jobs were advertised according to gender? And houses were rented according to race? Now access to jobs and housing (and to sexual expression) is available according to sexual preference/orientation: "House for rent: no swingers, please." "Federally funded job available: no gays, please."

WHAT'S A SEXUAL MINORITY?

As we look at this question, do keep in mind your experience with whatever minority you're most familiar: racial, ethnic, religious, and so forth. You'll see that "sexual minority" fits the familiar model of ethnic minority almost perfectly.

During three centuries of American history, "minorities" have included immigrants, Jews, African Americans, "Orientals," Mexicans, Quakers, Mormons, and Catholics. The designated "other" against which the majority defines itself, ethnic minorities have typically been described as:

- A homogeneous group
- Less than adult, perhaps even less than human
- Not "normal"
- Proselytizing or seducing "normal" people
- Dangerous and therefore needing to be controlled

- Practitioners of secret, exotic rituals
- Impulsive and/or compulsive

American society has historically maintained myths about minority groups, their activities, and the consequences of allowing minorities to follow their "nature." At the same time, society often lacks awareness about the extent to which minorities are deprived or in pain.

This is what it's like to be gay or bisexual in America, or to prefer sex that involves variations such as swinging, S/M, exhibitionism, cross-dressing, sex toys, or adult entertainment. The tens of millions of people in one or more of these categories know that their activities could cost them their job, their apartment, their physical safety, or their freedom at any time. They also know that anything that involves their sexuality may be met with ignorance, hostility, or both.

The way professionals are trained, and the services they provide us, are an example. To protect consumers by guaranteeing a minimum level of competence, all states credential professionals such as physicians, attorneys, and psychologists. Thus, everyone has the right to expect their doctor, lawyer, marriage counselor, social worker, and physical therapist to understand a variety of clients; lawyers are expected to understand that some children are cut out of their parents' wills. Physical therapists know that not everyone is right-handed.

When it comes to sexuality, training in all professions is limited, and many sexual minorities cannot expect expert or non-judgmental services. Because of lack of training and cultural ignorance/prejudice, a physician might misdiagnose an S/M-playing patient with bruises as an abuse victim (and be legally required to file a police report). A marriage counselor who doesn't understand open relationships might assume that a swinging couple coming for communication skills are afraid of intimacy. Many psychologists would mishandle a bisexual patient ambivalent about committing to marriage. Even Oprah's therapy guru, Dr. Phil, responded to a question about swinging with derision and ignorance. Calling a caller's boyfriend "a loser" and "slime," he cautioned her not to "whore yourself and screw his friends."[10]

One National Coalition for Sexual Freedom survey of those in alternate sexual lifestyles, for example, found that 30 percent of the respondents experienced discrimination, while 36 percent suffered violence or harassment (including losing jobs or custody of children).[11] A 2008 compilation of incident reports from thousands of men and women in alternate sexual lifestyles showed similar numbers.[12]

Similarly, Dr. Joseph Marzucco's 2004 study of 786 people regularly involved in sadomasochism showed that men and women were significantly concerned about getting adequate medical care if physicians saw the physical results of their sexual play.[13] The majority remain unknown to their physicians. With millions of Americans practicing S/M regularly or occasionally, studies like these reflect a serious public health problem.

A majority of women who self-identify as lesbians do not disclose their sexual behavior or orientation to their physicians. This can prevent them from receiving appropriate medical and psychological information and services.[14]

Let's turn now to some of the ways that sexual minorities—millions and millions of tax-paying, mind-their-own-business Americans—are facing legal and economic violence from judges, prosecutors, and other authorities.

"But blacks can't help being black," you might say, "while sexual expression is a choice, so a democratic society can pathologize any sexual choices it wishes." On the one hand, much sexual expression is inborn the same way race is. Sexual orientation—same-gender or other-gender—is, for almost everyone, fixed at birth or very early childhood. Millions of other people experience sexual preferences so strong that they function as an orientation. These can include sadomasochism, cross-dressing, exhibitionism, and a rigid erotic attachment to objects such as leather or rubber garments.

More to the point, America has also outlawed discrimination in employment and public accommodation based on a person's religion—which is adopted, not inborn. The right to wear a turban or cross in public is protected no matter how uncomfortable it makes others. There is no reason that someone's choice to go to a swing club can't be as protected as his or her choice to go to church (and yes, lots of Americans do both, swinging on Saturday night, praying on Sunday morning).[15]

CASE STUDY: CRIMINALIZING YOUR RIGHT TO SWING

Swingers' clubs—private places where couples and individuals can congregate and have sex with each other in a safe environment—have quietly existed in most major metropolitan areas (and many U.S. military bases) since the 1970s. Fueled by the aging of the baby boomer generation and their belief in personal liberty and sexual expression, the phenomenon has grown every decade since. By most estimates, there are now at least 5 million swingers in the United States.[16]

By 1966, the military had some 50,000 swingers in its ranks under investigation, and it intended to court martial and discharge all of them.[17] When civilian aerospace engineer Robert McGinley was identified as one of these "sexual deviants," he lost his Air Force security clearance (and therefore his job). In 1975, McGinley founded the Lifestyles Organization (LSO); in less than five years, LSO was hosting weekend conventions attended by 500 or more couples. Soon, hotels and resorts throughout southern California were bidding for their lucrative convention business. They had learned that these thousands of couples are relatively affluent, well-behaved, and often returned—with their friends. They were perfect customers.

But in 1996, some California state officials decided to discourage swinging and to "run LSO out of the state of California."[18] Since swingers weren't doing anything illegal, how could this be arranged? By declaring that their sexual behavior was dangerous: that it was immoral, which led to the breakdown of family values, and therefore bred crime. The police had no authority to stop this *legal* behavior, but the state did have an agency mandated to protect the "public morals" in places it licensed: the Department of Alcoholic Beverage Control (ABC).

And so, in October 1996, the ABC told the Seaport Marina Hotel in Long Beach that their liquor license could be revoked if they hosted the Lifestyles Halloween Banquet and Ball. Six weeks later, the ABC temporarily suspended the liquor license of the Town and Country Hotel in San Diego that had hosted the Lifestyles convention that August. In response, the hotel cancelled the contracts it had signed with LSO for the next three years.

A few months later, the ABC warned that any California hotel hosting the 1997 LSO convention (of 4,000 swingers) could lose its liquor license. ABC District Supervisor Dave Gill declared that their morality rules applied even at events at which no alcohol was served. Even more astonishing, he added that the ABC rules applied even to hotel sleeping rooms, since they were on the premises of license holders: "The regulations apply at all times to their facilities regardless of whether the activity is private or public in nature." The ABC was declaring that adults could not swing in their own locked hotel rooms. Frightened hotels and convention centers were breaking contracts with LSO left and right, creating financial havoc.[19]

In subsequent court hearings, the American Civil Liberties Union described the ABC as "drunk with its own power." Robert Burke, president of the University of California–Los Angeles Law School, accused the agency of practicing "state Gestapo-ism."[20] Ultimately, a 9th Circuit judge ruled that the ABC was aggressively misusing its authority in order to suppress expression, and he invalidated the regulations that prevented "any depiction of sex in any manner" at licensed venues. In addition, the ABC had paid the city of Long Beach to uncover dirt about LSO; the city was fined when it was discovered its police officers had lied about the debauchery they supposedly found while undercover at an LSO event.[21]

"From 1996–99, there were over 30,000 swing club gatherings in North America," reports multiple award–winning investigative journalist Terry Gould. "They were verifiably peaceful . . . I couldn't document a single 911 call placed from a club. But local police nationwide persisted in raiding these private clubs, arresting and humiliating couples inside. Sometimes tipping off TV stations ahead of time, police would drive people out into the glare of waiting cameras," he revealed in his landmark study, *The Lifestyle*. "Swinging is peaceful activity that the government insists on treating like criminal behavior."[22]

But the nationwide crackdown was just getting rolling.

You couldn't describe Phoenix as sleepy when the fuss there started, and you certainly wouldn't now—with a million and a half people, it's America's fifth largest city. By 1998, it had an active community of tens of thousands of swingers, with gay bathhouses, mixed-gender clubs, and regularly scheduled house parties. Lots of people got laid, and no one complained.

But then the Phoenix City Council adopted the Live Sex Act Business ordinance. Drafted primarily by the Christian-based National Family Legal Foundation, it declared that sex at a private swing club was a "live sex act," and that clubs are "detrimental to the health, safety and morals" of residents. It was adopted as an emergency ordinance so that the city could *declare* a problem rather than having to *prove* it. And so that the city could ignore the vocal input of "the community"—swingers.

The first U.S. law specifically banning swingers' clubs, the city's reasons for it were phony from the start:

- Eliminating prostitution, although not one complaint or arrest was ever made.
- Limiting overuse of police services, although no unusual level of calls was ever noted, and no one was ever arrested prior to the ordinance.
- Preventing STDs, although all clubs required safer sex practices, and no one has ever shown higher rates of STDs among swingers than among non-swingers. Not only did all clubs provide condoms, the gay club The Chute offered free HIV testing.[23]
- Preventing blight, although the clubs were in industrial and other non-glamorous neighborhoods. The building that housed The Chute was eventually sold for three times its original cost. Wouldn't you love to suffer such blight?
- Zoning infractions. The relentless, discriminatory inspections required club bathrooms to be cleaner than a restaurant's. Some inspectors promised to return daily. Clubs were cited for missing light bulbs.

Other problems the city's swing clubs and bathhouses never experienced were drunkenness, violence, guns, sexual assault, gambling, safety problems, financial irresponsibility, corruption, illegal drugs, or underage people. This is a record of public decorum unmatched by the Phoenix 7–Elevens or the Arizona State University football program.

And yet, ordinance in place, the Phoenix police hounded swing clubs. At a cost of millions of taxpayer dollars, they sent in undercover officers week after week (hazardous duty, to be sure—"Honey, it was all in the line of duty. I swear I didn't enjoy it."). When the busts came, it was by cops in riot gear, with guns drawn. Did they imagine the swingers had concealed weapons? It's hard to imagine a bunch of naked 40-year-olds in the middle of kissing, sucking, licking, and screwing becoming a dangerous mob. The night that police raided Flex, there were 10 felonies in the city including a car theft. It's a great example of how Phoenix's obsession with sex clubs distorted their public safety priorities.

Club owners spent hundreds of thousands of dollars in legal fees simply for the right to stay in business. They met with the city and attempted to compromise; the response was everything from bizarre applications of arcane hotel regulations ("no more than six in a bed") to falsified police reports. Courts disallowed documented facts while relying on the "common sense" of city and church officials, anonymous zoning inspectors, and reports by cops who perjured themselves. Phoenix City Attorney James Hays says he was instructed to do whatever was necessary to close down the clubs, especially the most elegant, Club Chameleon.

In 2002, a federal court ruled "there is no First Amendment protection for physical sexual conduct."

By 2005, the owners and staffs of six different clubs had been arrested and booked on charges ranging from facilitating live sex acts to "moral turpitude" (yes, really). They were told to expect serious jail time and large, punitive fines. Chute co-owner Donell McDonell was threatened with having to register as a sex offender for life. To lighten their sentences, most owners agreed to close their clubs (forfeiting their right to make a living). The very few that remained open were reduced to a desultory, cheap motel blandness, nothing like the vibrant joyfulness once enjoyed by so many. The sophisticated, non-violent, non-problematic Phoenix swing scene and bathhouse scene was destroyed.

And now, a decade after the ordinance's enactment? Couples still swing, and gay men still cruise. Except both groups do it in settings far less safe, less controlled, less healthy, and less dignified than they used to. "Some of the sex has moved to public parks," says McDonell bitterly, "probably with fewer condoms used. The Vice Squad says they're going after that next—having chased it there, from when it was safely behind our closed doors." "People are not going to stop what they are doing because there is no Club Chameleon," agrees former club owner Milo Fencl. "They'll find other ways to do what they want, even if they feel less comfortable with it."[24]

Legitimate business owners like the Fencls have learned that religious bigotry, not due process or ethical government, runs Phoenix. City Council members who helped push the discriminatory ordinance, like Peggy Bilstein, subsequently refused to discuss the matter, even if they were still on the City Council.

It's not just a bunch of gathering places that Bilstein, police lieutenant Larry Jacobs, and others shut down. An established community—with safety norms, etiquette, education, and mutual support, where people know and care for each other—was deliberately destroyed. "It was a place where women felt absolutely safe—they knew they were surrounded by people who would be respectful," laments Nancy Fencl, co-owner of the now-closed Club Chameleon.[25]

Phoenix didn't wipe out swinging. It just made swinging less safe, less predictable, less sober, less contained. All the things those in city government and the Community Defense Council sanctimoniously claimed they were worried about.

"The Phoenix ordinance is the first of its kind in this country," reported the *Phoenix New Times* in 1999, "and appears primed to spark a monumental battle in the legal war over the business of sex in America." How prescient. Cities that have criminalized swing clubs for consenting adults since 2004 include Philadelphia, Indianapolis, and St. Paul. The Community Defense Counsel (which is what the National Family Legal Foundation became) predicts many more cities will be cleansed.[26]

Contrast this situation with Canada's, which legalized swinging in 2005. Their Supreme Court used the exact opposite logic of American law:

"Criminal indecency or obscenity must rest on actual harm or a significant risk of harm to individuals or society," wrote Chief Justice Beverley McLachlin in the majority decision. "Consensual conduct behind code-locked doors can hardly be supposed to jeopardize a society as vigorous and tolerant as Canadian society."

The judge thus gave her fellow citizens the highest possible compliment.

As if responding to the main arguments threatening such clubs in the United States, the Canadian Court also said, "The causal link between images of sexuality and anti-social behavior cannot be assumed. Attitudes in themselves are not crimes, however deviant they may be or disgusting they may appear." And legalizing the clubs doesn't undermine the right to not go to them: "Only those already disposed to this sort of sexual activity were allowed to participate and watch," said the Court. The Court also dismissed the red herring of clubs spreading STDs. "Sex that is not indecent can transmit disease while indecent sex might not," they ruled.

But when it comes to sex, Americans have trouble seeing straight. Says Mayor Bart Peterson of Indianapolis, "Our zoning laws exist for a reason: to protect families and children from being exposed to the negative effects that adult businesses can have on a community. Illegal adult establishments like

Reel One are a detriment to strong, healthy neighborhoods and simply will not be tolerated in Indianapolis."[27] It isn't only swingers' gatherings that are attacked. S/M conventions have been harassed and disrupted by authorities around the country. Here are some recent examples:

- After N'awlins in November met in New Orleans annually without incident, police informed the host hotel that they'd be busted if it hosted the event again.
- When hotels in Maryland and Virginia notified police they would be hosting S/M events, alcohol control authorities threatened to suspend the hotels' licenses, even though no alcohol will be served there.
- San Diego; Baltimore; Washington, DC; and Attleboro, Massachusetts selectively enforce zoning and public indecency laws against local S/M communities.
- From February to May 2002 alone, S/M conventions were blocked by Concerned Women for America, American Family Association, and the American Decency Association. The coordinated media and civic attacks took place in Chicago, Oklahoma, St. Louis, and in Michigan.[28]

CASE STUDY: S/M

According to national surveys, 12 percent of American adults have engaged in consensual sadomasochism, erotic power play, or bondage-and-discipline games (S/M).[29] These sexual activities may or may not involve toys, equipment, and role-playing. They often involve physical stimulation that produces pain ranging from mild to intense. These games are always consensual, always negotiated ahead of time, and always accompanied by good communication skills and the ability to change or stop what's happening whenever desired.

Practitioners of alternative sexual lifestyles have not fared well in child custody hearings. Because America's family court system is often biased against sexual minorities, parties in divorce proceedings sometimes try to gain legal advantage by exposing a former partner's sexual history. Parental fitness has been questioned, for example, because one spouse has committed adultery, been "promiscuous," is gay, or participates in "unusual" sexual activity. Courts often agree, typically without evidence, that a child would be endangered because a parent engages in non-approved sexual behavior.

Over the years, I have been professionally involved in many custody proceedings that involved sexual issues. One of these was recently described in a peer-reviewed journal.[30] The article convincingly demonstrates how family courts can be prejudiced against sexual variations. It is noteworthy that this case took place in California, often considered the most sexually liberal and sexually educated state in the country. Here's the story.

When Mr. Smith and Ms. Smith divorced in the late 1990s, they shared custody of their son, Ed. The boy lived with his father; his mother had liberal visitation rights and alimony. Mr. Jones eventually became the mother's live-in boyfriend, whom everyone agreed soon had an excellent stepparenting relationship with Ed.

Years later, during an investigation about the boy's health (which was soon completed) when he was 11, Ms. Smith volunteered that she and Mr. Jones had an intense S/M relationship. This triggered an investigation about the fitness of the mother and the possible danger posed by the live-in boyfriend. The investigation (by court-appointed Dr. Blair) confirmed that:

- No child abuse had occurred.
- The child was unaware of the mother's sexual interests.
- The child never saw any incidents or suggestions of inappropriate sexual activity.
- The child was doing well emotionally and in school.

Nevertheless, Dr. Blair was concerned that the couple's interest in S/M would lead to dangerous or illegal activities. He stated that Mr. Jones had a sexual interest in children but admitted that there was no evidence to support this belief. Despite this, he said Mr. Jones could pose a risk to Ed in the future. Dr. Blair admitted there was no evidence that the couple was ignorant or careless, but he worried about "the effects on the child if Ms. Smith were to die or become impaired during sexual activity."[31]

Worse still, Dr. Blair decided that the couple's consensual sexual activities constituted domestic violence. And while noting that "the child has not observed it," Dr. Blair wildly speculated that "he is exposed to the after-effects," even though "I don't have enough information to understand what the effects on the child might be."[32]

As a result of Dr. Blair's alarm and recommendations, the court severely limited the mother's visitation and custody rights, ended her alimony, and required her to attend psychotherapy for almost a year—specifically focusing on domestic violence. The court ended Ed's relationship with Mr. Jones, even though all parties agreed Ed had a better relationship with him than with his biological father. All of this, despite Dr. Blair's opinion that the boy was well-adjusted and healthy.

It is heartbreakingly ironic that, although victims of domestic violence rarely have their children taken from them, the court's insistence on treating Ms. Smith as a victim of domestic violence provided the rationale for limiting her contact with her own child. According to the National Coalition for Sexual Freedom, there are hundreds of tragic cases like this every year. Says national forensic expert Dr. Charles Moser, "We know of no cases where the parent admitting to S/M interests obtained or retained custody of the minor."[33] America's family courts are directed to act in the best interests of the children they see. Ignorance about sexual behavior, whether S/M, bisexuality, non-monogamy, or anything else, can make it impossible for courts to fulfill this mandate.

CASE STUDY: PREVENTING YOUR RIGHT TO LEARN AND DISCUSS

In April 2009, sex educator Megan Andelloux began the process of leasing office space in the Grant Building in Pawtucket, Rhode Island. Her goal was to create an educational institution open to the public, The Center for Sexual Pleasure and Health (CSPH). "We'd have seminars and discussion groups, a library, guest speakers, training for professionals, it would be great," she said.

Five months of investment, preparation, and publicity followed. And three days before the CSPH was slated to open on September 26, 2009, the city of Pawtucket told Andelloux that city councilmembers and city officials had received an e-mail reading, "Hello, A center for 'sexual rights' and 'sexual pleasure' is opening in Pawtucket."[34] In response, the city blocked the Center's opening.

The city said it couldn't allow the CSPH to open because of zoning codes. Although the building was zoned for multi-purpose uses, zoning director Ronald Travers said the allowed uses included only business, entertainment, restaurant, office, or personal use. "There is no provision for educational use, so I had to deny the applicant," interpreted Travers.

City administrator Harvey Goulet, Jr. admitted that he and some other city officials objected to the CSPH's mission. "I would prefer that it not be in Pawtucket. That's my opinion and that's the mayor's opinion," he said. "I think some of these things would be better off in an office somewhere than a storefront." Convenient rumors began rumbling: that the CSPH would be a brothel, a center for sex trafficking, and an abortion clinic—all demonstrably untrue (if only because the rented space was less than 550 square feet). The opposition feared the community talking openly about sexuality, and some powerful people were using their political muscle to prevent legal educational activities and speech with which they were uncomfortable.

Andelloux contested the zoning interpretation, especially because the Grant Building housed other "educational" businesses, including a chess academy. The CSPH formally appealed the city decision and was again denied occupancy, which brought in the Rhode Island ACLU. Executive director Steven Brown said, "The city's intent is to suppress the speech that would otherwise occur at the Center. Such content-based discrimination raises serious constitutional concerns."

After threatening court action, Andelloux applied for a special use permit in January 2010. The Pawtucket appeal board eventually awarded CSPH a special use permit, and the Center opened on February 2, 2010—more in debt than it expected, although with correspondingly more publicity.

* * *

Compassionate Americans look back in shame at the distorted rulings that historically mar our otherwise proud legal system. Decisions involving runaway slave Dred Scott, the Japanese internment camps, legalized racial segregation, and the denial of women's right to vote fill us with wonder: "What were those judges thinking?" The time will come when our descendants look back on the routine denial of child custody to capable, caring parents who happen to make love the "wrong" way or to the "wrong" gender, and they will wonder the same thing about us.

GAY AMERICANS

According to every study of American sexual behavior, at least 25 million heterosexual men and women have same-gender sex one or more times in their adult lives. Not surprisingly, they remain straight.

About 8 million Americans have sex with people of the same gender throughout their adult lives. Like everyone else, most of these Americans fall in love at some point. And like everyone else, they want to be left alone to go to work, raise their kids, pay their bills, and watch TV. They're not looking for approval, just the chance to live a decent life. And they want their basic rights—visiting their partner in the hospital, handling their kids' school stuff, keeping their job even though their boss hates "fags."

That's it. That's the whole gay thing.

But some people are obsessed with homosexuality, seeing it as a poison that must be stopped. They talk about protecting themselves and their loved ones from the evil Gay Agenda. Here, for example, is the guiding principle behind the American Family Association's (AFA) opposition to this alleged Gay Agenda:

We oppose the efforts of the gay movement to force its agenda in education, government, business and the workplace through law, public policy and the media . . . We oppose the effort to convince our culture that because individuals participate in homosexual behavior, they have earned the right to be protected like racial and other minority groups.[35]

But the AFA has it wrong. It isn't having gay sex that earns you protection in America. It's being American. That's why blacks and Mormons and people with handicaps are "protected"—because they're American. That's all that gays want—the normal protections of all Americans.

So besides wanting "protection," what is this Gay Agenda?

"Middle America better take note. Last night Hollywood exposed its own corrupt agenda. [It] is no doubt on a mission to homosexualise America," said Stephen Bennett of Straight Talk Radio, after the 2006 Golden Globe Awards honored films like *Brokeback Mountain* and *Capote*.[36]

What does that even mean? If Bennett thinks gays are lined up around the block to have sex with him, he's flattering himself. Are gays determined to seduce straights? Of course not. Do they want to destroy marriage? No, they cherish it so much, they want to join it themselves (unlike millions of straight people, abandoning it in droves). But not because they want the cake, the dress, or the flowers. They want the civil rights. Yes, every state is in the marriage business, and it awards financial, legal, and parenting rights to married people. That's what gay Americans want—the "special rights" the government gives the people it marries.

How would this affect anyone else's marriage? In Massachusetts, the only state that allows same-sex marriage, the heterosexual divorce rate has *gone down*. Some would chide that gay marriage helps *protect* "traditional" marriage. No one's marriage is threatened by same-sex marriage any more than your friendships are threatened by mine. Nevertheless, in 1996, Congress passed the Defense of Marriage Act (DOMA), which defines marriage as a legal union between one man and one woman; it prevents the federal government from recognizing the validity of legal same-sex marriages, and it allows states to *not* recognize same-sex marriages that are legal in another state.

As if this weren't enough, in 2006 twenty-nine U.S. senators took time out from fighting global terrorism, our declining education system, and skyrocketing health care costs to sponsor a Constitutional amendment that would prevent any state from allowing same-gender marriage "or the legal incidents thereof" (those "special rights" gay people want).[37]

The Republican Party would soil our beautiful Constitution by pandering to some of its constituents' worst fears. "When America's values are under attack, we need to act," said then–Senate Majority Leader Bill Frist (R-TN). Apparently he meant the American "value" of discrimination.

This legal discrimination already exists in a range of parenting arenas, such as child custody (gays lose it) and adoption (difficult or against the law). Referring to the fact that some states allow same-sex couples to adopt children, radio host Janet Parshall told Larry King, "[I] think what you have in many respects is state-sanctioned child abuse."[38] Would Larry King have sat there quietly if she had said this about adoption by black or Jewish parents?

Not that it will change any minds, but there are dozens of published psychological and sociological studies showing that children of gay parents do just as well as children of heterosexual parents.[39]

Christian conservatives say that homosexuality offends God. (They mean, of course, *their* god.) I am perfectly willing to believe that—but so what? Lots of what we do in the United States offends their God. working on the Sabbath, heterosexual adultery, embezzlement, drinking alcohol, blasphemy. None of these is illegal in the United States, because "offending God" isn't a crime.

So why should homosexuality be legally disadvantaged, just because some people don't like who some other people have sex with? The fundamental agreement in America law is that simply offending others' beliefs will never be illegal. That's rule number one: "Life, liberty, and the pursuit of happiness."

The Family Research Council (FRC) says that once people are allowed to marry someone of the same gender, they will want the right to marry animals. Yes, they really said that. It's impossible to say how many of their leaders or followers really believe that, but it's part of the systematic lies and distortions of the Religious Right. Along with Focus on the Family, Concerned Women for America, and other groups, FRC's goal is to scare people.[40]

The real story is that the Republican Party has decided to mobilize Christian believers. Since communism is dead, and terrorism apparently doesn't scare people enough, homosexuality is the most frightening thing they can think of. Karl Rove predicted that putting an anti-gay measure on the 2004 Ohio ballot would bring millions of new evangelical voters to the polls, and it worked perfectly, reelecting George Bush. Blaming liberal, urban, young, sex-crazed homosexuals for the fear, alienation, depression, and powerlessness that average Americans feel (as the direct result of Bush's policies) may be bad karma but it's smart politics. Having persuaded conservative Christians that gays want to steal their country, Republicans are promising to protect them from this insidious threat.

And since the government and Religious Right are already waging a War on Sex, the civil rights of gays and other sexual minorities can be just one more front, one more casualty-strewn battleground.

This is one way in which the War on Sex is part of something bigger and far more sinister.

Chapter Fifteen

REVOLUTIONIZING AMERICAN GOVERNMENT—BAD NEWS FOR DEMOCRACY

If adult entertainment has so many customers, why is there so little outcry when these businesses are harassed, chased out of town, or closed? Why don't customers hold elected city councils, state assemblies, and local judges accountable? Why don't they challenge uninformed local churches, lying civic groups, and biased media?

Adult entertainment is a textbook example of the limits of democracy and the tyranny of the loud. Since local institutions do typically respond to pressure, a vocal minority can shut down what a majority won't speak up about. That's why it's so crucial that everyone agree on the basic rules of fair governance, an agreement that does *not* exist in America when it comes to sexuality. Certain rights are so fundamental that they must *not* be put up for a vote. A majority should not have the right to strip the minority of its rights, a danger that both Alexis de Tocqueville and John Stuart Mill foresaw almost two centuries ago.

Most people aren't shy about revealing the kind of car they drive; if the state legislature proposed to ban Toyotas, satisfied Toyota owners would make a fuss. Similarly, most people will tell you their favorite food, and if it were suddenly subject to a huge tax or limits on availability, its devotees would squawk.

But despite the size of its audience, adult entertainment patrons are not eager to reveal their interests. We live in such a sex-negative environment that adult customers around the country are shamed and demonized; few

Americans are willing to lose their job or marriage simply to keep the local strip club open.

Since patronizing adult businesses is typically a hidden activity, no one can support it in the normal open way that true democracy requires. Customers won't write letters to the editor, complain to their city councilman, or educate their clergy. And so, realistically, supporting the rights of adult entertainment can be done only (1) in principle and (2) by outside organizations. Opponents of adult businesses exploit this by claiming *they* speak for the community, pretending that they don't know that the community is full of customers and supporters who feel intimidated about speaking out—upstanding taxpayers and parents like us.

Opponents of adult entertainment typically focus on denying a *business's* right to function, to "just make money" and "degrade" sexuality. They rarely mention their *neighbors'* rights to consume this entertainment. Citizens for Community Values, for example, says adult businesses "prey upon unsuspecting towns, cities, and counties that don't have [preventive] legislation in place, in order to open their 'sex-for-sale' establishments."[1] You'd think these businesses were kidnapping unwilling townspeople and forcing them to watch the "sex for sale." This is the same manipulative strategy that focuses on denying "pornographers'" rights without discussing *consumers'* rights, attempting to limit broadcasters' rights without discussing *viewers'* rights, and eliminating "abortionists'" rights without discussing *patients'* rights.

A naïf might imagine that if only the consumers of adult material would reach a critical mass, they would become a political force, but if that were true, it would have happened already. Millions of Americans already go to swing clubs, and tens of millions more patronize strip clubs, massage parlors, adult bookstores, nude beaches, home sex toy parties, X-rated DVDs, and other forms of adult entertainment. But the social sanction against such activities is so strong that almost no one will stand up and defend what he or she does, much less assert its wholesomeness.

Democracy isn't working because one side (anti-pluralism and pro-censorship) represents cultural (although not behavioral) normativity, while the other side (consumers of adult materials) suffers with cultural dystonia (typically involving shame, guilt, and silence). In an environment so ambivalent and negative about sexuality, the typical individual will deny and fear his or her eroticism. So when the civic subject is in any way related to sexuality, any pro-sex voice dies in the throat. This civic paralysis means that sex-positive individuals will always be dramatically marginalized. It will be almost impossible to gather the momentum needed to reach the threshold of political influence—of *civic visibility.*

And so one group, the Parents Television Council (PTC), can generate over 98 percent of all indecency complaints to the Federal Communications

Commission (FCC) over the course of two years (and via a mechanical e-mail blaster, at that). As senior research fellow at George Mason University's Mercatus Center Adam Thierer notes, the PTC is quickly acquiring a "heckler's veto" over programming in America, as many of the shows they complain about receive significant fines or are even driven off the air.[2]

But virtually no one writes to the FCC outraged that same-gender kissing is forbidden on network television 24 hours per day; no one complains when shows are tortured with bleeps and electronic gauze. The FCC received very few complaints that the Rolling Stones were muzzled during their 2006 Super Bowl halftime performance—exactly as they had been on the *Ed Sullivan Show* 40 years earlier. And when something with sexual authenticity sneaks in—Chris Rock on Comedy Central, a condom machine in a nightclub bathroom, the cleavage parade on Oscar night, a pharmacy that carries emergency contraception without a fuss—sex-positive people are pleased to remain invisible, rather than enjoying a moment out of the closet and telling *someone*, "Yes, this works for me. I like living in this world. Thank you."

Seventy years after its founding, America was torn by one of the bloodiest civil wars the world had ever seen. Both sides fought like they understood it was a war for the soul of the nation. One hundred fifty years after that, we again face a profound conflict about the soul of our nation. Will it be a secular, pluralist democracy as the Founders envisioned, or a theocratic, authoritarian one like the lands they left behind?

Those who war on sex often remind us that the Founders wanted everyone to worship as he or she desired. They leave out a crucial detail—the Founders wanted no institution forcing or shaping that worship. Today's War on Sex is a struggle over whether institutions will have the right to force Americans to worship—to conform to a single vision of "morality," "chastity," "decency," "family values," even "faith."

When the Civil War ended in 1865, boys and men from each side wearily embraced and shared what little food there was. They stopped to worship their common God and talked about planting their common crops. In years to come, these former enemies would gather together on the Gettysburg battlefield and embrace again, marveling at how they had changed each others' lives forever.

I don't see us doing this again for many generations, if ever. Those who war on sex mistrust my vision of individual autonomy, sexual integrity, faith in pluralism, and tolerance of differences. They hate what they perceive as our arrogance, narcissism, hubris, and dependence on reason rather than fear. They particularly resent living in a world that will not let them completely run away from their sexual impulses and crippling guilt.

Democracy, secularism, and pluralism are messy, scary, and inefficient— unlike theocracy or totalitarianism. This radical system requires people to accept being periodically uncomfortable as the price for the benefits they get from it (benefits that start with one's own choices being tolerated by everyone else). When people are no longer willing to manage their discomfort about others' choices, our entire system breaks down.

We can see the early stages of this in America today, where some people don't believe they have to accept their own discomfort about others' choices.[3] They frame their rejection of this civic requirement as their religious obligation, *but they are breaking the democratic covenant.* You can see the resulting polarization of Americans and American politics, as a significant portion of the public is attempt to delegitimize—not disagree with, but delegitimize—the decisions and rights of the rest of the country. We're all in trouble as a result.

What, then, will be the basis for public policy: fact, science, and personal autonomy, or faith, a single morality, and anxiety reduction? This is *the* central question in world politics today. The fact that the vehicle for America's internal discourse is sexuality shouldn't lull us into thinking we're dealing with something trivial.

We're not.

EPILOGUE: ONE BRIGHT SPOT

While Americans of all age, educational, and political groups have continued to suffer with the results of the War on Sex, there is one bright spot. Since the first edition of this book was published, lesbians and gay men have made great strides toward legal equality with non-gay Americans.

Ironically, it is the political will of one of American society's most marginalized groups that is not only gaining itself equal rights but is simultaneously keeping the door open for sexual rights for all people during an otherwise dark time. Here are some highlights—some victories in America's War on Sex:

- Americans are more supportive of gay people and issues than ever before. In 2011, 56 percent of Americans considered same-sex relations to be "morally acceptable"—up from only 40 percent a decade earlier.[1] In 2010 and 2011, six national polls found majority support for marriage equality.[2] Polls show continued increases in the support of gay families, and a majority of Americans now support equal job opportunities, benefits, and access to leave for gay men and lesbians in the workplace.
- In 2011, New York became the sixth state to legalize same-gender marriage (as does the District of Columbia); eight others offer civil unions to committed couples, conferring many spousal rights.[3] The federal government announced it will no longer defend the discriminatory Defense of Marriage Act (DOMA) (see Chapter 14), enraging many who somehow fear the effect of same-gender marriage on

mixed-gender marriage. At this time, there are still 12 U.S. states that have voted to prohibit same-gender marriage.

- Religious denominations are increasingly welcoming gay Americans. In 2011, the Presbyterian Church (U.S.A.) approved the ordination of homosexual clergy, joining Episcopalians, Unitarians, several other Christian denominations, and most Jewish denominations that also ordain gay and lesbian clergy.
- The Gay-Straight Alliance movement—student-run clubs in high schools (and some colleges)—has evolved in 33 states, involving at least 40,000 students and dozens of high-profile celebrities. While these clubs raise consciousness about homophobia and bullying of gay kids, they simultaneously normalize and humanize homosexuality for straight kids. And they provide a place for all participants to talk about sexual feelings and questions without fear of judgment or punishment—something badly missing in many schools, homes, and churches.
- In 2010, a new federal policy was announced allowing unmarried gay partners to visit their loved ones in the hospital.
- For the first time, gay Americans can finally serve openly in the military. After almost two decades of hypocrisy and persecution, the shameful "Don't Ask, Don't Tell" law was finally overturned in late 2011. Gay men and lesbians are now free to protect America alongside their straight countrymen and -women.

To tell the truth, I feel safer already.

NOTES

FOREWORD

1. See *Loving v. Virginia*, 388 U.S. 1 (1967). (The Court struck down, in a lawsuit brought by the ACLU, anti-miscegenation laws that were still on the statute books in 16 states.)

2. Lindsey Gruson, "Second Thoughts on Moments of Silence in the Schools," *New York Times*, March 4, 1984, sec. 6E.

3. See for example, Thomas Jefferson, "Eternal vigilance . . . ," *QuoteDB*, http://www.quotedb.com/quotes/2283 (April 13, 2006).

4. *Lawrence v. Texas*, 539 U.S. 558 (2003); *Romer v. Evans*, 517 U.S. 620 (1996).

5. See, for example, *Ashcroft v. American Civil Liberties Union*, 542 U.S. 656 (2004); *Ashcroft v. American Civil Liberties Union*, 535 U.S. 564 (2002); *Ashcroft v. Free Speech Coalition*, 535 U.S. 234 (2002); *United States v. Playboy Entertainment Group*, 529 U.S. 803 (2000); *Reno v. American Civil Liberties Union*, 521 U.S. 844 (1997).

6. *Lawrence v. Texas*, 539 U.S. 558 (2003).

7. *Bowers v. Hardwick*, 478 U.S. 186 (1986).

8. John Bartlett, *Bartlett's Familiar Quotations*, ed. Justin Kaplan (Boston: Little, Brown, and Company, 1992), 643.

9. John Stuart Mill, *On Liberty* (Indianapolis: Hackett, 1978 [1859]), 73.

10. See note 6 above, 562.

11. See, for example, *Nebraska Press Ass'n v. Stuart*, 427 U.S. 539, 582 (1976); *Smith v. California*, 361 U.S. 147, 169 (1959).

12. See note 6 above.

13. See note 6 above, 590.

14. *Brown v. Board of Education*, 347 U.S. 483, 74s.ct. 686 (1954).

15. *Planned Parenthood v. Casey*, 505 U.S. 833 (1992).

16. See note 15 above, 851.

17. President, American Civil Liberties Union; Professor of Law, New York Law School. For research assistance with this Foreword, Professor Strossen gratefully acknowledges Steven Cunningham (NYLS '99) and Brenna Sharp (NYLS '07).

INTRODUCTION

1. Obama predicted he would do this in his 2006 book, *The Audacity of Hope*.

2. http://pewresearch.org/pubs/971/both-mccain-and-obama-favor-expanding -faith-based-initiatives.

3. http://www.politicususa.com/en/alliance-defense-fund-attacks-law-banning -churches-from-politicking.

4. http://www.youtube.com/watch?v=xIC_vc8YOj4.

CHAPTER ONE

1. http://www.rhrealitycheck.org/blog/2011/09/07/birth-control-will-create-pagan -society-based-consequencefree.

CHAPTER TWO

1. Hannah Brückner and Peter Bearman, "After the Promise: The STD Consequences of Adolescent Virginity Pledges," *Journal of Adolescent Health* 36, no. 4 (2005): 271–78.

2. www.religioustolerance.org/abonbr.htm.

3. Judith Levine, *Harmful to Minors: The Perils of Protecting Children from Sex* (Minneapolis: University of Minnesota Press, 2002), 90.

4. Dozens of lectures in various U.S. locales, 1980–2000.

5. Debra Hauser, "Five Years of Abstinence-Only-Until-Marriage Education: Assessing the Impact," *Advocates for Youth*, http://www.advocatesforyouth.org/ PUBLICATIONS/stateevaluations.pdf, 5.

6. Scott Williams, "Abstinence Becomes a Business," *Milwaukee Journal Sentinel*, October 9, 2000. sec. 510(B) (abstinence-only program funding alone supports more than 700 programs nationwide); See also, Peggy Burch, "Just Say 'Not Yet' Lecturer Pushes 'Sexual Revolution'—Abstinence," *The Commercial Appeal*, October 14, 2000, sec. G1 (describing the "Aim for Success" abstinence-only program, a family business that runs abstinence-only education programs in schools in eight states).

7. Sexuality Information and Education Council of the United States, "SIECUS State Profiles: A Portrait of Sexuality Education and Abstinence-Only-Until-Marriage Programs in the States Released Today," *SIECUS*, March 23, 2005, http://www.siecus.org/media/press/press0095.html.

8. The World Health Organization and other researchers agree that, over a period of a year, about 99 percent of the uninfected partners of "always" condom users

remained HIV negative. BBC News, "Condoms: The Science," *BBC News*, June 27, 2004, http://news.bbc.co.uk/1/hi/programmes/panorama/3845011.stm.

9. National Center for HIV, STD and TB Prevention, Division of HIV/AIDS Prevention, "HIV/AIDS among Men Who Have Sex with Men," July 2005. *Department of Health and Human Services, Centers for Disease Control and Prevention*, July 2005, http://www.cdc.gov/hiv/PUBS/Facts/msm.htm.

10. Abstinence Clearinghouse, "Take the Condom Quiz," brochure available from http://www.abstinence.net.

11. Matt Apuzzo, "Study: Abstinence May Lead to Risky Acts," *SFGate.com*, March 18, 2005, http://sfgate.com/cgi-bin/article.cgi?file=/news/archive/2005/03/18/national/a115514S47.DTL.

12. See http://www.silverringthing.com.

13. "The Pledge," on *60 Minutes*. First broadcast May 22, 2005 by CBS.

14. Ibid.

15. U.S. House of Representatives, Committee on Government Reform, Minority Staff, Special Investigations Division. *The Content of Federally Funded Abstinence-Only Education Programs*, prepared for Representative Henry A. Waxman (Washington, DC: Government Printing Office, 2004), http://www.democrats.reform.house.gov/Documents/20041201102153–50247.pdf.

16. Clara S. Haignere, Rachel Gold, and Heather J. McDaniel, "Adolescent Use of Condoms and Abstinence: Are We Sure We Are Teaching What Is Safe?" *Health Education and Behavior* 26, no. 1 (1999): 43–54.

17. Marty Klein, "Government Report: Abstinence Programs Lie," *Sexual Intelligence*, January 2005, http://www.sexualintelligence.org/.

18. Of course, the whole Bush administration was anti-science: global warming, pollution, overfishing, Plan B, and so forth. In 2004, the government's own CDC Web site ignited a firestorm with its deliberate inaccuracies about sexual health. In 2005, it even tried to appoint a veterinarian to head the Women's Health Division of the FDA. Today's national Republican Party (including the Tea Party) continues this anti-science legacy.

19. Bill Frist, speech at the Health Legacy Partnership (HELP) conference, Washington, DC (October 22, 2003).

20. See note 1 above.

21. http://mathematica-mpr.net/publications/pdfs/impactabstinence.pdf

22. Professional Data Analysts, Inc. and Professional Evaluation Services, "Minnesota Education Now and Babies Later Evaluation Report 1998–2002," as prepared for the Minnesota Department of Health, January 2004.

23. Peter Bearman and Hannah Brückner, "Promising the Future: Virginity Pledges and the Transition to First Intercourse," *American Journal of Sociology* 106, no. 4 (2001): 859–912.

24. See note 1 above.

25. Marty Klein, "Virginity Pledges >>STDs," *Sexual Intelligence*, April 2005, http://www.sexualintelligence.org/newsletters/issue62.html#four.

26. "For Many, Abstinence Doesn't Work," *Sexual Intelligence*, August 2003, http://www.sexualintelligence.org/.

27. Committee on Economic, Social and Cultural Rights, 22nd session. *General Comment 14. The Right to the Highest Attainable Standard of Health*, Paras. 12(B), 16 and Note 8, 2000, http://hrw.org/reports/2002/usa0902/USA0902–07.htm#P729 _181328.

28. www.aolnews.com/2010/04/07/wis-da-threatens-arrest-for-local-sex-ed -teachers/. See also http://www.jsonline.com/news/statepolitics/90020507.html.

29. http://www.whec.com/article/stories/S2246779.shtml?cat=0?video=YHI&t=a.

30. http://www.familiesaretalking.org/index.cfm?fuseaction=Feature.showFeature &FeatureID=2034.

31. Committee on Economic, Social and Cultural Rights, 22nd session. *General Comment 14. The Right to the Highest Attainable Standard of Health*, Paras. 12(B), 16 and Note 8, 2000, http://hrw.org/reports/2002/usa0902/USA0902–07.htm#P729 _181328. *General Comment 24(52), General Comment on Issues Relating to Reservations Made Upon Ratification or Accession to the Covenant or the Optional Protocols Thereto, or in Relation to Declarations Under Article 41 of the Covenant*, U.N. Human Rights Committee, 52nd sess., 1989, para. 11; and *General Comment 14. The Right to the Highest Attainable Standard of Health*, Committee on Economic, Social and Cultural Rights, para. 12(b) and note 8.

32. See *General Comment 14. The Right to the Highest Attainable Standard of Health*, Committee on Economic, Social and Cultural Rights, paras. 12(b), 16 and note 8.

33. *General Comment 24(52), General Comment on Issues Relating to Reservations Made Upon Ratification or Accession to the Covenant or the Optional Protocols Thereto, or in Relation to Declarations Under Article 41 of the Covenant*, U.N. Human Rights Committee, 52nd sess., 1989, para. 11.

34. Office of the United Nations High Commissioner for Human Rights and the Joint United Nations Programme on HIV/AIDS, "HIV/AIDS and Human Rights-International Guidelines" (from the Second International Consultation on HIV/AIDS and Human Rights, Geneva, September 23–25, 1996), U.N. Doc. HR/PUB/98/1, Geneva, 1998, para. 38(h).

35. "Conclusion," in *Ignorance Only: HIV/AIDS, Human Rights and Federally Funded Abstinence-Only Programs in the United States, Human Rights Watch 14, no. 5* (September 2002), http://hrw.org/reports/2002/usa0902/USA0902-08.htm#P796 _199849.

CHAPTER THREE

1. Jerry Falwell, "The Moral Majority Coalition," *Jerry Falwell Ministries,* http://www.falwellsecure.com/libertyalliance/otgh/.

2. http://www.alliancedefensefund.org/Home/ADFContent?cid=4690.

3. http://www.myfoxhouston.com/dpp/news/politics/100209-texas-constitution -governor.

4. CWA Mission Statement, http://www.cwfa.org/content.asp?ID=18226.

5. http://www.rightwingwatch.org/content/ken-cuccinelli-hosting-concerned -women-america-fundraiser.

CHAPTER FOUR

1. The Planned Parenthood Federation of America, "The Assault on Birth Control and Family Planning: Executive Summary" (New York: The Planned Parenthood Federation of America, 2003), 2.

2. Senator Richard Durbin speaking on the floor of the Senate on the Partial-Birth Abortion Ban Act of 2003, March 11, 2003, S3469.

3. As Pope Benedict said in his first encyclical, "Monogamous marriage" is on a par with "the image of a monotheistic God." The pope notes that "marriage based on exclusive and definitive love becomes the icon of the relationship between God and his people and vice versa." Heterosexual romantic love is described as "the one in particular [that] stands out [from all other love] . . . where body and soul are inseparably joined and human beings glimpse an apparently irresistible promise of happiness." See, Rocco Palmo, "The Surprising Message Behind 'God Is Love,'" *Beliefnet*, 2006, http://beliefnet.com/story/184/story_18403_1.html.

4. "Evangelicals and STDs," *SexInfo*, http://www.soc.ucsb.edu/sexinfo/ ?article=stds&refid=039.

5. It also raises the standard of living for entire countries. See the ongoing work of International Planned Parenthood Federation (http://www.plannedparenthood.org) and the Alan Guttmacher Institute (http://www.guttmacher.org/).

6. Shulamith Firestone, *The Dialectic of Sex: The Case for Feminist Revolution* (New York: Morrow, 1970).

7. Although the Catholic hierarchy had trouble accepting test-tube babies at first, and a few radicals still reject artificial insemination.

8. K. Greenwood, and L. King, "Contraception and Abortion," in *Women in Society*, ed. Cambridge Women's Studies Group (London: Virago, 1981).

9. Patricia Spallone, "Reproductive Technology and the State: The Warnock Report and its Clones," in *Made to Order: The Myth of Reproductive and Genetic Progress*, ed. Patricia Spallone and Deborah Lynn Steinberg (Oxford: Pergamon), 173–74.

10. Ann Friedman, "Over-the-Counter Insurgency," *Mother Jones*, November 29, 2005, http://www.motherjones.com/news/update/2005/11/planb_timeline.html.

11. James Dobson, "HPV Epidemic Plagues Young People," *Focus on the Family*, uExpress, January 12, 2003, http://www.uexpress.com/focusonthefamily/index.html ?uc_full_date=20060108.

12. Ibid.

13. Marty Klein, "FDA Bad-Mouths Condoms," *Sexual Intelligence*, December 2005, http://www.sexualintelligence.org/newsletters/issue70.html#four.

14. Associated Press, "Debate Ranges over Condom Labeling," *FOXNews.com*, June 29, 2005, http://www.foxnews.com/story/0,2933,160981,00.htm.

15. Henry J. Kaiser Family Foundation, "Vatican Continues to Debate Condom Use to Prevent HIV Transmission, Church Leaders, Theologians Say," *The Body: The Complete HIV/AIDS Resource*, March 22, 2004, http://www.thebody.com/kaiser/ 2004/mar22_04/vatican_condoms.html.

16. http://www.guttmacher.org/statecenter/spibs/spib_MWPA.pdf.

17. http://www.guttmacher.org/media/inthenews/2011/07/13/index.html.

18. Boonstra HD et al., *Abortion in Women's Lives* (New York: Guttmacher Institute, 2006).

19. B. Major et al., *Report of the Task Force on Mental Health and Abortion, American Psychological Association, Task Force on Mental Health and Abortion, 2008*, Washington, DC, http://www.apa.org/pi/wpo/mental-health-abortion-report.pdf.

20. The Planned Parenthood Federation of America, "Planned Parenthood Sues to Protect South Dakota Women," *Planned Parenthood*, June 6, 2005, http://www.plannedparenthood.org/pp2/portal/media/pressreleases/pr-050606-abortion.xml.

21. http://www.guttmacher.org/pubs/MandatoryCounseling.pdf.

22. http://www.theatlantic.com/national/archive/2011/03/free-speech-hypocrisies-of-pro-lifers/72868/.

23. Guttmacher Institute, State Policies in Brief, "Mandatory Counseling and Waiting Periods for Abortion," *Guttmacher Institute*, May 1, 2006, http://www.guttmacher.org/statecenter/spibs/spib_MWPA.pdf.

24. Center for Reproductive Rights, "2005 Mid-Year Report," *Center for Reproductive Rights*, 2005, http://www.crlp.org/st_leg_summ_midyear_05.html.

25. http://www.guttmacher.org/pubs/fb_induced_abortion.html.

26. R. K. Jones and K. Kooistra, "Abortion Incidence and Access to Services in the United States, 2008" *Perspectives on Sexual and Reproductive Health* 43, no. 1 (2011): 41–50.

27. Ibid.

28. The Abortion Access Project, "Fact Sheet: The Shortage of Abortion Providers," *The Abortion Access Project*, http://www.abortonaccess.org/newpages.php?id=6.

29. http://www.catholicsforchoice.org/topics/healthcare/documents/2005factsabout catholichealth care.pdf.

30. http://www.mergerwatch.org/ec-in-the-er/ about the NON-use of EC in ERs for rape victims.

31. Megan Cooley, "Catholic Hospitals Refuse Patients Contraception," *Women's eNews*, February 4, 2003, http://www.womensenews.org/article.cfm/dyn/aid/1209.

32. http://www.catholicsforchoice.org/topics/healthcare/documents/2002 secondchancedenied_001.pdf.

33. B. A. Robinson, "Abortion and Roman Catholic Hospital Mergers," *ReligiousTolerance.org*, December 8, 2000, http://www.religioustolerance.org/abo _rcc.htm.

34. http://www.stlouisreview.com, August 30, 2002.

35. *San Jose Mercury-News*, October 13, 2011, P.B6.

36. Gary Heinlein, "Bill Would Ban Over-Counter Sales of Morning-After Pill: As FDA Examines Nonprescription Sales of Drug, a State Lawmaker Aims to Ward Off Its Widened Use," *Detroit News Online*, November 25, 2005, http://www.det -news.com/apps/pbcs.dll/article?AID=/20051125/POLITICS/511250337/1003/ METRO.

37. The Unborn Victims of Violence Act (also known as "Laci and Conner's Law"), signed into law by President George W. Bush on April 1, 2004.

38. According to studies by the FDA and National Abortion Federation, there are no known long-term risks associated with using mifepristone and misoprostol.

Feminist Women's Health Center, "The Abortion Pill: Mifepristone and Misoprostol for Early Abortion,"*Feminist Women's Health Center*, October 25, 2005, http://www.fwhc.org/abortion/medical-ab.htm.

39. Lynn M. Paltrow, "Prison or Rehab: What Is the Best Place for a Pregnant Woman Using Illicit Drugs?" *ReconsiDer: Forum on Drug Policy*, http://www.reconsider.org/asp/biography.asp?SpeakerID=1501; *Ferguson v. City of Charleston*, 532 U.S. 67 (2001).

40. http://www.guardian.co.uk/world/2011/jun/24/america-pregnant-women-murder-charges.

41. http://www.personhoodusa.com/what-is-personhood.

42. Guttmacher Institute, State Policies in Brief, "Refusing to Provide Health Services," *Guttmacher Institute*, February 1, 2006, http://www.guttmacher.org/statecenter/spibs/spib_RPHS.pdf.

43. Adam Sonfield, "New Refusal Clauses Shatter Balance between Provider 'Conscience,' Patient Needs," *Guttmacher Report on Public Policy* 7, no. 3 (August 2004), http://www.guttmacher.org/pubs/tgr/07/3/gr070301.html.

44. http://aksarbent.blogspot.com/2011/10/nebraska-social-workers-want-referrals.html.

45. Adam Sonfield, "New Refusal Clauses Shatter Balance between Provider 'Conscience,' Patient Needs," *The Guttmacher Report on Public Policy* 7, no. 3 (August 2004), http://www.guttmacher.org/pubs/tgr/07/3/gr070301.html.

CHAPTER FIVE

1. http://www.drjudithreisman.com/archives/2005/12/senate_subcommi.html.

2. http://alturl.com/xz73a.

3. http://commerce.senate.gov/public/index.cfm?p=Hearings&ContentRecord_id=e8088f9f-d8d2-4e82-b012-46337c6f9456&Statement_id=d744db10-1a94-4899-a3ea-fcf5cf0d6493.

4. http://www.boston.com/bostonglobe/ideas/articles/2008/07/20/abducted/?page=full.

5. http://thinkprogress.org/politics/2009/05/07/39152/robertson-child-molestation/.

CHAPTER SIX

1. Brent Bozell, Parents Television Council, http://www.parentstv.org/ptc/community/speech.htm.

2. In *Lawrence v. Texas*, 539 U.S. 558 (2003).

3. "Dick Cavett and Comedy on the Streets," *San Jose Mercury News*, May 4, 1994. Also at http://www.bookreporter.com/community/quote/02-09.asp, at September 1.

4. Advocates for Youth, "European Approaches to Adolescent Sexual Behavior & Responsibility," *Advocates for Youth*, 2006, http://www.advocatesforyouth.org/news/events/stdytour.ht

5. For a non-nude example of a sexy European TV commercial that would not be aired in America, see http://www.break.com/cute-girls/WTF-European -Commercial-387387.html.

6. The Parents Television Council, "Comedy Central Roast Brings Unspeakable Vulgarity into Two-Thirds of American Homes," *PTC Insider* 7, no. 10 (October 2005) http://www.parentstv.org/ptc/publications/insider/2005/October.pdf.

7. *The 60th Annual Golden Globe Awards*, first broadcast January 19, 2003 by CBS. Directed by Chris Donovan and Al Schwartz.

8. See Timothy Taylor, *The Prehistory of Sex* (New York: Bantam, 1997).

9. Mary Calderone, conversation with author, spring 1987.

10. http://www.youtube.com/watch?v=Lt70kMn7O9s.

11. *Butler v. Michigan* (1957).

12. The whole question of what the relevant "community" is in the Internet age now begs for a different, modern answer. See http://www.nytimes.com/2008/06/24/ technology/24obscene.html and http://www.lawrencewalters.com/site-articles/ digital-age/.

13. Michael Scherer, "The FCC's Cable Crackdown," *Salon.com*, August 30, 2005, http://archive.salon.com/news/feature/2005/08/30/fcc_indecency/index_np .html.

14. Robert Corn-Revere, "Can Broadcast Indecency Regulations Be Extended to Cable Television and Satellite Radio?" *Progress on Point* 12, no. 8 (May 2005), http://www.pff.org/issues-pubs/pops/pop12.8indecency.pdf.

15. Censorship crusader Senator Ted Stevens (R-AK), among others, is using the same justification to restrict programming on cable TV. See his congressional "decency" hearings, for example, March 11, 2005, http://www.sfgate.com/cgi-bin/ article.cgi?file=/n/a/2005/03/01/national/w141707S29.DTL.

16. Motion Picture Production Code of 1930, articles 1, 2, and 3, www .artsreformation.com/a001/hays-code.html.

17. James R. W. Bayes, Kathleen A. Kirby, and Martha E. Heller, "Third Circuit Court of Appeals Revisits Earlier Decision on Media Ownership Rules," Wiley Rein & Fielding LLP, October 2004, http://www.wrf.com/publication_newsletters.cfm ?ID=11&year=2004&publication_ID=9525&keyword=].

18. Marjorie Heins, personal e-mail to author, April 17, 2006. See also her media democracy fact sheet at http://www.fepproject.org/factsheets/mediademocracy.html.

19. Kevin J. Martin, Letter to Parents Television Council concerning f-word decision, December 5, 2003, http://www.parentstv.org/PTC/fcc/2003/martin -letter2.htm.

20. http://www.theorator.com/bills108/hr3717.html.

21. Michael Hayes, "Bush Signs Indecency Bill, Fines for Broadcasters Increase Tenfold," *Xbiz News*, June 16, 2006, http://xbiz.com/news_piece.php?id=15545.

22. Notable exceptions are Emancipation, Prohibition, and criminalizing contraception.

23. James Poniewozik, "The Decency Police," *Time Archive*, March 28, 2005, http://www.time.com/time/archive/preview/0,10987,1039700,00.html.

24. Jeff Jarvis, "The Shocking Truth About the FCC: Censorship by the Tyranny of the Few," *BuzzMachine*, November 15, 2004, http://www.buzzmachine.com/archives/2004_11_15.html.

25. http://www.janetjacksonflash.com/.

26. http://www.parentstv.org/PTC/news/release/2009/0220.asp.

27. http://www.liberty.edu.

28. Todd Shields, "FCC Hires Conservative Indecency Critic," *Mediaweek*, August 8, 2005, http://www.mediaweek.com/mw/news/recent_display.jsp?vnu _content_id=1001010563.

29. Penny Nance, on *Fox News Live* with Bob Sellers, July 19, 2004. See http://www.mediamatters.org/items/200407200005.

30. See note 28 above.

31. Ibid.

32. Ben Scott, http://www.americanprogress.org/site/pp.asc?c=biJRJ80VF &b=480225.

33. *New York Times*, December 30, 1969.

34. http://www.parentstv.org/ptc/familyguide/main.asp.

35. Ben Charney, "Janet Jackson Still Holds TiVo Title," *CNETNews.com*, September 29, 2004, http://news.com.com/Janet+Jackson+still+holds+TiVo+title/2100-1041_3-5388626.html.

36. CNN Newsnight Aaron Brown, "Debate over FCC Guidelines," *CNN.com*, November 17, 2004, http://transcripts.cnn.com/TRANSCRIPTS/0411/17/asb.01 .html.

37. For example, see the mission statement of Morality in Media, at http://www .moralityinmedia.org/.

38. The video is produced by the We Are Family Foundation. http://www .wearefamilyfoundation.org/; "SpongeBob, Barney Promote 'Gay' Agenda? 61,000 Schools to Receive 'We Are Family' Video with Lesson Plan," *WorldNetDaily*, January 6, 2005, http://www.worldnetdaily.com/news/article.asp?ARTICLE _ID=42253.

39. Cary Wiggins, http://meetingthesinlaws.com.

40. Personal communication, October 17. 2011.

41. See note 13 above.

CHAPTER SEVEN

1. Rob Garver, "The Family Research Council Says Anti-clerical Judges Pose a Greater Danger Than Al-Qaeda," *The American Prospect Online Edition*, April 13, 2005, http://www.prospect.org/web/page.ww?section=root&name=ViewWeb &articleId=9499.

2. "Chapter VII. Discrimination Based on Gender and Sexual Orientation," in *Ignorance Only: HIV/AIDS, Human Rights and Federally Funded Abstinence-Only Programs in the United States, Human Rights Watch* 14, no. 5 (September 2002), http://hrw.org/reports/2002/usa0902/USA0902-06.htm.

3. National Abortion Federation, "Bush's Strategy to Restrict Reproductive Freedom: A Chronology," *National Abortion Federation*, 2005, http://www.prochoice.org/policy/national/bush_strategy.html.

4. Advocates for Youth, "Will the Politics of Teen Sex Stop a Cancer Vaccine?" *Advocates for Youth*, 2005, http://www.advocatesforyouth.org/publications/cancervaccine.htm.

5. Tad Walch, "Family Group Draws BYU into Porn Fray," *DeseretNews.com*, September 25, 2003, http://deseretnews.com/dn/view/0,1249,515034237,00.html.

6. Ken Tucker, "Station Pulls Keillor for 'Offensive Content'," *Billboard Radio Monitor*, August 12, 2005, http://billboardradiomonitor.com/radiomonitor/news/business/net_syn/article_display.jsp?vnu_content_id=1001014255.

7. Parents Television Council, "Frequently Asked Questions," *Parents Television Council*, 2004, http://www.parentstv.org/PTC/faqs/main.asp#Arent%20you%20violating%20First%20Amendment%percent20freedoms%20by% 20censoring%20TV%20shows.

8. Daniel Weiss, "Porn Feeds Human Trafficking," *DenverPost.com*, January 27, 2006.

9. Jerry Falwell, "The Moral Majority Coalition," *Jerry Falwell Ministries*, http://www.falwellsecure.com/libertyalliance/otgh/.

10. House Government Reform Committee, Subcommittee on Criminal Justice, Drug Policy and Human Resources, *CDC's Human Papillomavirus (HPV) and Cervical Cancer Prevention Activities*, March 11, 2004.

11. Brian Skoloff, "Ave Maria Co-Founder Backs Off Moral Stance," *HeraldToday.com*, March 5, 2006, http://www.bradenton.com/mld/bradenton/news/local/14019307.htm?source=rss&channel=bradenton_local.

12. "President Bush Signs Unborn Victims of Violence Act of 2004: Remarks by the President at Signing of the Unborn Victims of Violence Act of 2004," *The White House*, April 1, 2004, http://www.whitehouse.gov/news/releases/2004/04/20040401-3.html.

13. CNN Larry King Live, "Debate over Gay Marriage," *CNN.com*, January 17, 2006, http://transcripts.cnn.com/TRANSCRIPTS/0601/17/lkl.01.html.

14. "U.S. Senate Judiciary Committee Hearing on Judge Samuel Alito's Nomination to the Supreme Court, Part II of II," *WashingtonPost.com*, January 9, 2006, http://www.washingtonpost.com/wp-dyn/content/article/2006/01/09/AR2006010901016.html.

15. Nick Farrell, "Watching Web Porn Is 'Cheating'," *VnuNet.com*, June 12, 2002, http://www.vnunet.com/vnunet/news/2119054/watching-web-porn-cheating.

16. Abstinence Clearinghouse, "First Lady Laura Bush Endorses Abstinence," *Abstinence Clearinghouse*, January 18, 2006, http://www.abstinence.net/library/index.php?entryid=2480.

17. Diane, "Culture of Fear, Culture of Death," *ToughEnough.org*, May 22, 2005, http://toughenough.org/2005/05/culture-of-fear-culture-of-death.html.

18. Morality in Media, et al., Letter to President George W. Bush re Supreme Court nominee, July 14, 2005, http://www.obscenitycrimes.org/news/Bush_letter_re_Sup_Ct_nominee_(Jul05).pdf.

19. Tom Strode, "Life Digest: Mass. To Promote Destructive Stem Cell Research; Calif. Reconsiders Assisted Suicide; S.D. Pro-Life Bills Now Law," *BPNews.net*, April 4, 2005, http://www.bpnews.net/bpnews.asp?ID=20511.

20. "Is Sex Ever Really 'Safe'?" Focus on the Family, http://www.troubledwith.com/stellent/groups/public/@fotf_troubledwith/documents/articles/twi_013892.cfm?channel=Parenting %Teens&topic=Sexual%Activity&sssct=Background%20Info.

21. Oppose Censorship in Omaha, "Censorship in Omaha," *Oppose Censorship in Omaha*, January 2005, http://www.omaha-neb.com/censorship.html.

22. Nicholas A. Jackson, "Public Libraries, the Left, and the Corruption of Children," *The Conservative Voice*, August 8, 2005, http://www.theconservativevoice.com/articles/article.html?id=7377.

23. Jane Lampman, "Churches Confront an 'Elephant in the Pews'," *The Christian Science Monitor*, August 25, 2005, http://www.csmonitor.com/2005/0825/p14s01-lire.html.

24. "The Pledge," in *60 Minutes*, first broadcast May 22, 2005 by CBS.

25. http://www.youtube.com/watch?v=tdeIZmg2Sxw.

26. http://thefire.org/spotlight/codes/220.html.

27. http://www.cbsnews.com/stories/2004/03/11/national/main605394.shtml.

28. http://www.youtube.com/watch?v=-R0GYhsX-o8&NR=1.

29. http://moralityinmedia.org/full_article.php?article no=45.

30. http://www.rightwingwatch.org/content/kern-doubles-down-claim-homosexuality-more-dangerous-terrorist-attacks

31. http://www.damemagazine.com/dame-daily/features/f261/AlabamavsDildos.php?PageId=1.

32. http://www.personhoodusa.com/press-release/ohio-reaches-first-milestone-personhood-amendment-drive

33. http://www.politico.com/news/stories/0411/53314.html.

34. http://www.texastribune.org/texas-politics/2010-texas-governors-race/gov-rick-perry-on-abstinence-sanctuary-cities

35. http://www.rightwingwatch.org/content/fischer-homosexual-agenda-americas-greatest-immediate-threat

36. http://caffeinatedthoughts.com/2011/10/interview-with-rick-santorum-a-champion-for-the-family-manufacturing-jobs/

37. http://articles.latimes.com/2008/nov/05/nation/na-scotus5.

38. Peter Lattman, "Justice Alito's Thank You Note to James Dobson," *The Wall Street Journal Online*, March 2, 2006, http://blogs.wsj.com/law/2006/03/02/justice-alitos-thank-you-note-to-james-dobson/.

CHAPTER EIGHT

1. The federal government also spent *millions* of dollars on such operations in 2005; for example, on pursuing and prosecuting Edward Wedelstedt of Littleton,

Colorado, for operating a chain of adult video arcades. See http://www.free speechcoalition.com/wedlestedtsentenced1.htm.

2. Larry Walters, personal phone call with author, October 14, 2011.

3. *City of Erie v. Pap's A.M.*, 529 U.S. 277 (2000).

4. Officials in San Bernardino, California, are trying to blur the distinction between prostitution and erotic dancing in an obvious attempt to close local strip clubs. The local district attorney alleges that women dancers are having sex with each other in front of men who pay to watch, which he says is prostitution. Since the California Penal Code describes prostitution as "any lewd act between persons for monies or other considerations," this legal strategy could actually succeed; Marty Klein, "Carpal Tunnel Censorship?" *Sexual Intelligence*, August 2000, http://www .sexualintelligence.org/newsletters/issue06.html#carpal.

5. San Antonio, Texas. See Marty Klein, *Sexual Intelligence: An Electronic Newsletter*, Issue 59, January 2005, www.SexualIntelligence.org/newsletters/issue59 .html#five.

6. *Renton v. Playtime Theatres*, 457 U.S. 41 (1986).

7. Dissenting in *Boos v Berry*, 485 U.S. 312 (1988).

8. Three years later, Antonin Scalia said the same thing in attempting to uphold Texas's ban on sodomy in *Lawrence v Texas*, 539 U.S. 558 (2003).

9. The Free Expression Policy Project, "Fact Sheet on Sex and Censorship," *The Free Expression Policy Project*, http://www.fepproject.org/factsheets/sexand censorship.html.

10. *Flanigan's Enterprises, Inc. v. Fulton County, GA*, 00-11152, 11th Circuit, February 20, 2001.

11. *City of Los Angeles v. Alameda Books*, 535 U.S. 425 (2002).

12. S.B. No. 27 Sec. 4301.25 Section 3, http://www.legislature.state.oh.us/bills .cfm?ID=126_SB_27.

13. http://www.kmbc.com/news/29107173/detail.html#ixzz1b03KMB1e.

14. Mark Kernes, "The Myth of Secondary Effects," Free Speech Coalition, http://www.freespeechcoalition.com/Myth_of_Secondary_Effects.htm.

15. "Canadian Court Lifts Ban on 'Swingers' Clubs," *MSNBC.com*, http://www .msnbc.msn.com/id/10561253.

16. Richard Enrico, personal conversation with author, Fall 1989.

17. *City of Erie v. Pap's A.M.*, 529 U.S. 277 (2000).

18. http://www.ccv.org/About_CCV.htm.

19. Citizens for Community Values Web site/promotion.

20. For more on Burress's opportunistic collaboration with Karl Rove, see Chapter 14.

21. http://www.uaprogressiveaction.com/archives/2006/02/irs_delivers_wa.html.

22. Private correspondence with attorney, October 14, 2011. Name of attorney on file.

23. Val Walton, "ABC, Club Square Off over Topless Dancer Ban," al.com, November 1, 2005, http://www.al.com/news/birminghamnews/index.ssf?/base/ news/113084029965690.xml&coll=2.

CHAPTER NINE

1. George Lakoff, *Don't Think of an Elephant* (New York: Chelsea Green Publishing Company, 2004).

2. Marty Klein, *Sexual Intelligence*, Issue 30, August 2002, http://www.sexualintelligence.org/newsletters/issue30.html#five.

3. *Newsweek*, July 18, 2011, p.60

4. Nicholas A. Jackson, "Public Libraries, the Left, and the Corruption of Children," *Conservative Voice*, August 8, 2005, http://www.theconservativevoice.com/articles/article.html?id=7377.

5. Jan LaRue, "Let's End 'Victims of Pornography Month,' " *Morality in Media, Inc.*, 2004, http://www.moralityinmedia.org/index.htm?obscenityEnforcement/EndVOP-Month.htm.

6. Alan Leshner, personal conversation with author, June 3, 2003.

7. Robert Rector and Kirk A. Johnson, "Teenage Sexual Abstinence and Academic Achievement," *The Heritage Foundation*, October 27, 2005, http://www.heritage.org/Research/Welfare/whitepaper10272005-1.cfm, at footnote 1.

8. Steven Ertelt, "Planned Parenthood Abortions Increase, Now 20 Percent of U.S. Total," *LifeNews.com*, December 12, 2005, http://www.lifenews.com/nat1900.html; "Trends in Abortion in the United States, 1973–2002," The Alan Guttmacher Institute, January 2003, http://www.guttmacher.org/presentations/trends.pdf; Ceci Connolly, "Number of Abortion Providers at Its Lowest in Three Decades," *The Tech*, January 22, 2003, http://www-tech.mit.edu/V122/N65/Abortion.65w.html.

9. Daniel Patrick Moynihan, "Everyone has a right to. . .," BrainyQuote, http://www.brainyquote.com/quotes/authors/d/daniel_patrick_moynihan.html.

CHAPTER TEN

1. See Timothy Taylor, *The Prehistory of Sex* (New York: Bantam Books, 1996); and James Petersen and Hugh Hefner, *The Century of Sex* (New York: Grove Press, 1999).

2. Source for this list, unless noted, is Cindy Kuzma, "Sex and Technology: A Brief History" Planned Parenthood Federation of America, May 13, 2005, http://www.ppfa.org/pp2/portal/files/portal/webzine/artsculture/art-050513-sex-technology.xml.

3. Peter Johnson, "Pornography Drives Technology: Why Not to Censor the Internet" *Indiana Law*, 1997, http://www.law.indiana.edu/fclj/pubs/v49/no1/johnson.html.

4. See note 2, discussed in a phone call with *LibidoMag* editor Jack Hafferkamp, December 29, 2006.

5. WorldScreen.com, "TV Data: North America," *WorldScreen.com*, 2002, http://www.worldscreen.com/northamerica.php; See also note 3 above.

6. Oblivious to how these sexual uses made the now-valuable technology feasible for mass adoption in the first place.

7. David Sobel, "Internet Filters and Public Libraries," *First Amendment Center Publication* 4, no. 2 (October 2003),11, http://www.FirstAmendmentCenter.org/PDF/InternetFilters.pdf.

8. Center for Democracy & Technology, "Pennsylvania Web Blocking," Center for Democracy & Technology, 2004, http://www.cdt.org/speech/pennwebblock/.

9. For more information, see Bennett Haselton, *Peacefire.Org*, 2006, http://www.peacefire.org/.

10. "Internet Filter Review," *TopTenREVIEWS*, 2006, http://Internet-filter-review.toptenreviews.com/.

11. Bennett Haselton, e-mail to author, January 15, 2006.

12. Robyn Greenspan, "Porn Pages Reach 260 Million," *eSecurityPlanet.com*, September 25, 2003, http://www.esecurityplanet.com/trends/article.php/3083001.

13. Jonathan Wallace, "Federal Courts Use Censorware; Free Speech Advocates Object," The Censorware Project, 1998, http://censorware.net/reports/courtcen.html.

14. Karen Jo Gounaud, "Kids and the Internet: The Promise and Perils," *Testimony to the U.S. National Commission of Libraries and Information Science, Family Friendly Libraries*, http://www.nclis.gov/about/November-1988.pdf, page 105.

15. Sobel, 10.

16. Sobel, 9. According to their Web site, Family Friendly Libraries is affiliated with Focus on the Family and the Family Research Council.

17. Sobel, 10.

18. "A Briefing on Public Policy Issues Affecting Civil Liberties Online." *Center for Democracy & Technology Policy Post* 9, no. 12 (June 23, 2003), http://www.cdt.org/publications/pp_9.12.shtml.

19. Only California, New York, and Maine reject this federal money—specifically because they don't want Washington controlling their libraries.

20. *U.S. v. ALA*, 539 U.S. 194 (2003).

21. *U.S. v. ALA*, 539 U.S. 194, No. 02–361 (2003).

22. Will Doherty, "Sex and the Internet" (presentation to the Society for Scientific Study of Sexuality, San Jose, CA, April 12, 2003).

23. Doherty, "Sex and the Internet."

24. Bennett Haselton and Jamie McCarthy, "Blind Ballots: Web Sites of U.S. Political Candidates Censored by Censorware," *Peacefire.org*, November 7, 2000, http://www.peacefire.org/blind-ballots/.

25. See note 13 above.

26. Doherty, "Sex and the Internet."

27. Greg Lindsay, "Cybersitter Decides to Take a Time Out," *TIME Digital*, August 8, 1997, http://web.archive.org/web/20000830022313/http://www.time.com/time/digital/daily/0,2822,12392,00.html.

28. Doherty, "Sex and the Internet."

29. Xeni Jardin, "MSN Spaces: Seven Dirty Blogs," *Boing Boing*, December 2, 2004, http://www.boingboing.net/2004/12/02/msn_spaces_seven_dir.html.

30. *United States of America V. Robert Alan Thomas and Carleen Thomas*, F. App. 0032P (6th Cir.), Nos. 94-6648/6649 (1996), *Electronic Privacy Information Center*, http://www.epic.org/free_speech/censorship/us_v_thomas.html.

31. See note 18 above.

32. "A Briefing on Public Policy Issues Affecting Civil Liberties Online," *Center for Democracy & Technology Policy Post* 10, no. 14 (September 10, 2004), http://www.cdt.org/publications/pp_10.14.shtml.

33. 18 U.S.C. §2257.

34. See note 32 above.

35. http://articles.cnn.com/2009-04-07/justice/sexting.busts_1_phillip-alpert-offender-list-offender-registry?_s=PM:CRIME.

36. http://www.petaluma360.com/article/20110816/COMMUNITY/110819615/1362?tc=ix

CHAPTER ELEVEN

1. Despite terrorism, the miserable economy, and a crumbling infrastructure and education system, many people still cite homosexuality, abortion, teen sexuality, and pornography as America's central problems.

CHAPTER TWELVE

1. Barton Gellman, "FBI Forms Anti-Porn Squad; 'I Guess This Means We've Won the War on Terror,' One Agent Says," *SFGate.com*, September 21, 2005, http://www.sfgate.com/cgi-bin/article.cgi?file=/c/a/2005/09/21/MNGRSER4141.DTL&type=printable.

2. Ibid.

3. The case was *ABFFE v. Coakley;* I was one of the plaintiffs.

4. A key informant in this illegal bullying was Donald Wildmon, head of the then-new Religious Right pressure group, National Federation of Decency, which is now known as the powerful American Family Association. See Marjorie Heins, *Sex, Sin, and Blasphemy: A Guide to America's Censorship Wars* (New York: New Press, 1998), 70.

5. http://en.wikipedia.org/wiki/Melissa_Farley.

6. http://cybersolidaires.typepad.com/files/complaint-to-apa-against-mfarley.pdf.

7. http://www.afa.net/Detail.aspx?id=2147484055.

8. Jan LaRue, "What Are the U.S. Attorneys Doing for Victims of Pornography?" *Victims of Pornography*, 2004, http://www.victimsofpornography.org/Articles%20in%20The%20News/Articles%20in%20the%20News.htm.

9. Traditional Values Coalition, "The Plan to Win over Judicial Tyranny," *Our Battle Plan to Take Back Our Courts*, 2006, http://www.ourbattleplan.com/plan.php.

10. For example, on February 6, 2006, police seized more than *700* adult DVDs from Dr. John's Lingerie in Omaha, Nebraska, claiming they had *reason to believe* that *some* of the store's inventory violated state obscenity laws. "Dr. John" Haltom himself

was victimized by a number of raids at his store in Omaha, resulting in him serving several jail terms. See "Censorship in Omaha," *Oppose Censorship in Omaha*, January 2005, http://www.omaha-neb.com/censorship.html.

11. http://www.wired.com/politics/law/news/2005/08/68433 and http://www.taxfoundation.org/blog/show/1200.html.

12. "ASACP Data Indicates 99.9% of Validated CP Reports Are Not Related to Adult Entertainment Industry," Association of Sites Advocating Child Protection, *ASACP*, June 24, 2005, http://www.asacp.org/press/pr062405.html. http://www.asacp.org/whitepaper/ASACP-whitepaper-9-10-2010.pdf.

13. http://www.theatlantic.com/politics/archive/2011/08/the-legislation-that-could-kill-Internet-privacy-for-good/242853/.

14. As common as these allegations are, not a single one has ever been proven.

15. Nadine Strossen, *Defending Pornography: Free Speech, Sex, and the Fight for Women's Rights* (New York: Anchor Books, 1995), 299.

16. Such as the price of gasoline, the convenience of banking online, the luxury of not feeling uncomfortable at the beach, and the comfort of not being faced with too many questions about sexual things from one's children.

17. http://www.wired.com/science/discoveries/news/2004/11/65772.

18. *American Library Ass'n. v. Thornburgh*, 713 F. Supp. 469 (D.D.C. 1989).

19. Civil action 05-CV-01126-WDM-BNB.

20. 983 F.2d 248, 250 (DC Cir. 1990); 965 F.2d 8484 (10th Cir. 1992).

21. See note 11 above.

22. Eugene Volokh, "Obscenity Crackdown—What Will the Next Step Be?" *CATO Institute*, April 12, 2004, http://www.cato.org/tech/tk/040412-tk.html.

23. From the government's subpoena, reported in Howard Mintz, "Feds After Google Data," *MercuryNews.com*, January 19, 2006, http://www.siliconvalley.com/mld/siliconvalley/13657386.htm.

24. *Gonzales v. Google, Inc.* (2006), can be found at "The Internet and the Law," *Find Law*, http://news.findlaw.com/hdocs/docs/google/gonzgoog11806m.html.

25. Cameron W. Barr, "Policing Porn Is Not Part of Job Description: Montgomery Homeland Security Officers Reassigned after Library Incident," *Washington Post.com*, February 17, 2006, http://www.washingtonpost.com/wp-dyn/content/article/2006/02/16/AR2006021602066.html.

26. I am indebted to Alan Soble for a remarkable discussion of this concept in his book. Alan Soble, *Pornography, Sex, and Feminism* (Amherst, NY: Prometheus Books, 2002).

27. See also Marty Klein, "The Meaning of Sex," http://sexed.org/archive/article03.html.

28. That's one part of what makes obscenity trials so bizarre. A jury of strangers sitting fully clothed in a conference room watches porn to determine what it means to the so-called average person (whoever that is). How can their experience possibly relate to the experience of watching the film at home, in private, naked, playing with a consenting partner or masturbating alone?

29. Personal conversation with Web site owner "Igor," September 1, 2011.

30. As sex educator Dr. Sol Gordon used to say, "guilt can provide the energy for the repetition of behavior people feel conflicted about."

CHAPTER THIRTEEN

1. In America, various indecency statutes still criminalize blasphemy and moral turpitude. At least the punishments involve fines and prison rather than death

2. Dan Bilefsky, "Denmark Is Unlikely Front in Islam-West Culture War," *NYTimes.com*, January 8, 2006, http://select.nytimes.com/search/restricted/article ?res=FA0D12FC34540C7B8CDDA80894DE404482.

3. BBC News, "Mass Anti-Cartoon Rally in Beirut: Hundreds of Thousands of Shia Muslims in Lebanon Have Turned a Religious Ceremony into a Protest over Cartoons Satirising the Prophet Muhammad," *BBC News*, February 9, 2006, http://news.bbc.co.uk/1/hi/world/middle_east/4697286.stm.

4. See http://www.personhoodusa.com.

5. *Planned Parenthood v. Casey*, 505 U.S. 833 (1992).

6. Richard John Neuhaus, "A Voice in the Relativistic Wilderness: The Pope Crusaded For "Moral Truth." We Should Welcome His Help," *ChristianityToday.com*, April 4, 2005, http://www.christianitytoday.com/ct/2005/109/44.0.html.

7. Ibid.

8. Richard Owen, "Limbo Consigned to History Books," *Times Online*, November 30, 2005, http://www.timesonline.co.uk/article/0,13509–1897480,00.html.

9. Boethus says this in his The Consolation of Philosophy; see Kenneth Humphreys. "Putting the Dark into the Dark Age: 'Wonderful Events That Testify to God's Divine Glory," *Jesus Never Existed*, 2004, http://www.jesusneverexisted.com/dark-age.htm; for Tertullian, see David King, "Chapter 9: Religion," in *A Guide to the Philosophy of Objectivism*, http://rous.redbarn.org/objectivism/Writing/DavidK-ing/GuideToObjectivism/CHAPTR09.HTM.

10. "President Bush Signs Unborn Victims of Violence Act of 2004: Remarks by the President at Signing of the Unborn Victims of Violence Act of 2004," *The White House*, April 1, 2004, http://www.whitehouse.gov/news/releases/2004/04/20040401–3.html; See also National Abortion Federation, "Bush's Strategy to Restrict Reproductive Freedom: A Chronology," *National Abortion Federation*, 2005, http://www.prochoice.org/policy/national/bush_strategy.html.

11. Joshua Green, "Roy and His Rock," *Atlantic Online*, October 2005, http://www.theatlantic.com/doc/200510/roy-moores-ten-commandments.

12. Thomas B. Edsall, "Christian Right Mobilizes for Judge: Conservative Tilt Sought on Bench," *WashingtonPost.com*, January 9, 2006, http://www.washingtonpost.com/wpdyn/content/article/2006/01/08/AR2006010801069.html.

13. Laurie Goodstein, "Minister, a Bush Ally, Gives Church as Site for Alito Rally," *NYTimes.com*, January 5, 2006, http://select.nytimes.com/gst/abstract.html ?res=FB0B14F63A540C768CDDA80894DE404482.

14. Ronald Stoddart, director of Nightlight Christian Adoption, Washington, DC, May 24, 2005.

15. http://www.pfaw.org/pfaw/general/default.aspx?oid=17625.

CHAPTER FOURTEEN

1. http://www.sexualintelligence.org/newsletters/issue34.html.

2. "Church Passes the Plate for County Fight," Free Speech X-Press, February 10, 2006, http://www.freespeechcoalition.com/FSCview.asp?coid=301.

3. http://advanceindiana.blogspot.com/2005/08/four-star-general-fired-for.html.

4. Portions of Justice Scalia's dissent appeared in Judge Vaughn Walker's 2010 ruling in *Perry v. Schwarzenegger* supporting same-sex marriage and finding California's Proposition 8 unconstitutional.

5. See Marty Klein, *Your Sexual Secrets: When to Keep Them, When and How to Tell* (New York: Dutton, 1988).

6. Many commentators were shocked, *shocked* that men and women told Kinsey they enjoyed such "perversions" as oral sex, premarital sex, and anal sex. One of the main reasons his two best-selling volumes were damned after publication in the late 1940s and 1950s—*and continue to be damned*—is that some people don't want to know that so-called normal people actually do these things.

7. Julia Heiman, personal e-mail to author, fall 2005.

8. From memo written by Judy Guerin, Executive Director, National Coalition for Sexual Freedom, December 6, 2001, 2.

9. Robert Peters, "The Link between Pornography and Violent Sex Crimes," *Morality in Media*, 2004, http://www.moralityinmedia.org/index.htm?pornsEffects/Porn-Crime-Link-RWP.htm.

10. Marty Klein, "Oprah and Dr. Phil: Sex for the Simpleminded," *Playboy*, January 2003, 33–34; Also available at http://sexed.org/archive/article18.html.

11. National Coalition for Sexual Freedom, "Violence and Discrimination Survey," *National Coalition for Sexual Freedom*, 1999, http://www.ncsfreedom.org/library/viodiscrimsurvey.htm.

12. https://ncsfreedom.org/resources/bdsm-survey/2008-bdsm-survey-fast-facts.html.

13. Joseph Marzucco, "Healthcare Attitudes of Individuals in the Alternative Sexual Lifestyle; Bondage and Discipline, Sadism and Masochism," unpublished study, 2005.

14. The Planned Parenthood Federation of America, "For the Record: Lesbian, Gay, Bisexual, Transgender, Questioning (LGBTQ)," *Planned Parenthood*, 2006, http://www.plannedparenthood.org/pp2/portal/files/portal/webzine/ontherecord/otr-archive-lgbtq.xml.

15. Friendship Express, "What Is Swinging?" 1994, http://friendshipexpress.com/SWINGING.HTM. Data gathered by private swing clubs indicate that 90 percent of swingers identify a religious preference and 47 percent regularly attend religious services (Friendship Express, 1994; Miller, 1994; also Gould, 1999).

16. See, Terry Gould, *The Lifestyle: A Look at the Erotic Rites of Swingers* (Toronto, Ontario: Random House, 1999), 392. This is confirmed in various survey data.

17. I am indebted to Terry Gould for bringing this investigation and other details to public attention in *The Lifestyle* (see note 16 above).

18. Robert McGinley, phone call with author, February 20, 2006.

19. Dave Gill and others ultimately lost their jobs for criminally overreaching their mandate. (See note 18 above.)

20. See note 15 above.

21. See note 18 above.

22. See note 16 above.

23. Actually, heterosexual swingers' demographics and lifestyle make them one of the lowest risk groups for STDs, especially HIV. See Gould, 1999; Richard J. Jenks, "Swinging: A Review of the Literature," *Archives of Sexual Behavior* 27, no. 5 (1998): 507–21.

24. Milo Fencl, personal conversation with the author, November 10, 2005.

25. Nancy Fencl, personal conversation with the author, November 10, 2005.

26. David Holthouse, "Civil Libertines: The Battle over Phoenix's Groundbreaking Sex-Club Ban Moves into Federal Court," phoenixnewtimes.com, March 18, 1999, http.//www.phoenixnewtimes.com/issues/1999–03–18/feature2.html.

27. Sex Blog, "US Judge Orders Sex Club to Shut Down," *Salon.com*, May 28, 2005, http://blogs.salon.com/0003915/2005/05/29.html.

28. National Coalition for Sexual Freedom, "History of the NCSF: Hard at Work to Defend Your Rights," *National Coalition for Sexual Freedom*, May 2003, http://www.ncsfreedom.org/history.htm.

29. Sam Janus and Cynthia L. Janus, *The Janus Report on Sexual Behavior* (New York: Wiley, 1993): xiii, 430.

30. Marty Klein and Charles Moser, "S/M (Sadomasochistic) Interests as an Issue in a Child Custody Proceeding," *Journal of Homosexuality* 51, no. 3 (2006): 233–42. Note that participants' names are changed to protect anonymity.

31. Ibid.

32. Ibid.

33. Ibid, p. 240

34. The e-mail was sent by University of Rhode Island professor Donna Hughes. It didn't mention that Hughes had recently sponsored a campaign to make Rhode Island's prostitution laws stricter, and that Andelloux had testified against the campaign in a Rhode Island Senate hearing. See http://thecsph.org/about/history-of -the-csph/

35. Austin Cline, "Religious Right: AFA, Position on Homosexuality." *About.com*, http://atheism.about.com/library/FAQs/rr/blfaq_rr_afa_homosexuality.htm.

36. "Hollywood Sinks to New, All-Time Moral Low to 'Homosexualize' America," *Straight Talk Radio*, January 17, 2006, http://www.earnedmedia.org/sbm0117.htm.

37. The amendment was written by the Alliance for Marriage, with the assistance of Judge Robert Bork and other constitutional conservatives. The organization wants to make marriage more important, and divorce more difficult to obtain.

38. CNN Larry King Live, "Debate over Gay Marriage," *CNN.com*, January 17, 2006, http://transcripts.cnn.com/TRANSCRIPTS/0601/17/lkl.01.html.

39. For example, N. Andersen, C. Amlie, and E. A. Ytteroy, "Outcomes for Children with Lesbian or Gay Parents: A Review of Studies from 1978 to 2000," *Scandinavian Journal of Homosexuality* 43, no. 4 (2002): 335–51; S. Dundas and

M. Kaufman, "The Toronto Lesbian Family Study," *Journal of Homosexuality* 40, no. 2 (2000): 65–79.

40. Timothy J. Dailey, "The Slippery Slope of Same-Sex 'Marriage'," *Family Research Council*, http://www.frc.org/get.cfm?i=BC04C02&f=WA06B27.

CHAPTER FIFTEEN

1. Citizens for Community Values, "Sexually Oriented Businesses," CCV.org, http://www.ccv.org/What_is_a_Sexually_Oriented_Business.htm.

2. Adam Thierer, "Of *Desperate Housewives* and Desperate Regulators," http://www.cato.org/tech/tk/050105-tk.html.

3. As noted previously, we can see the same process occurring in Western Europe, where fundamentalist Muslims do not accept the necessity of managing their discomfort about their neighbors' behavior and speech.

EPILOGUE

1. Gallup, "Values and Beliefs," 2011. Cited in The Momentum Report—2011 Edition, published by the Movement Advancement Project. Report accessed at http://www.lgbtmap.org/file/momentum-report-2011.pdf.

2. CNN Opinion Research Poll, August 11, 2010; CBS News Poll, October 2010; ABC News/Washington Post Poll, "Gay Marriage," March 2011; CNN Poll, April 2011; Public Religion Research Institute, "Religion and Politics Tracking Survey," May 2011; Gallup, "Values and Beliefs Poll," May 2011. Cited in The Momentum Report—2011 Edition, published by the Movement Advancement Project. Report accessed at http://www.lgbtmap.org/file/momentum-report-2011.pdf.

3. http://www.ncsl.org/default.aspx?tabid=16430.

SELECTED BIBLIOGRAPHY

Collins, Ronald, and Sam Chaltain. *We Must Not Be Afraid to be Free*. New York: Oxford University Press, 2011.

Elias, James, et al., eds. *Porn 101: Eroticism, Pornography, and the First Amendment*. Amherst, NY: Prometheus Books, 1999.

Gould, Terry. *The Lifestyle*. Toronto: Random House, 1999.

Harvey, Philip. *The Government vs. Erotica*. Amherst, NY: Prometheus Books, 2001.

Heins, Marjorie. *Not in Front of the Children: "Indecency," Censorship, and the Innocence of Youth*. New York: Hill and Wang, 2001.

Heins, Marjorie. *Sex, Sin, and Blasphemy*. New York: The New Press, 1998.

Herdt, Gilbert, ed. *Moral Panics, Sex Panics*. New York: New York University Press, 2009.

Horowitz, Helen Lefkowitz. *Rereading Sex*. New York: Vintage Books, 2002.

Kincaid, James. *Erotic Innocence: The Culture of Child Molesting*. Durham, NC: Duke University Press, 1998.

Kipnis, Laura. *Bound and Gagged: Pornography and the Politics of Fantasy in America*. Durham, NC: Duke University Press, 1999.

Lane, Frederick. *The Decency Wars*. New York: Prometheus, 2006.

Levine, Judith. *Harmful to Minors*. Minneapolis, MN: University of Minnesota Press, 2002.

Lynn, Barry. *Piety and Politics: The Right-Wing Assault on Religious Freedom*. New York: Harmony, 2006.

Morone, James. *Hellfire Nation*. New Haven, CT: Yale University Press, 2003.

Petersen, James, and Hugh Hefner. *The Century of Sex*. New York: Grove Press, 1999.

Ryan, Christopher, and Cacilda Jetha. *Sex At Dawn*. New York: HarperCollins, 2010.

Soble, Alan. *Pornography, Sex, and Feminism.* Amherst, NY: Prometheus Books, 2002.

Strossen, Nadine. *Defending Pornography.* New York: New York University Press, 2000.

Taverner, Bill, and Sue Montfort. *Making Sense of Abstinence.* Morristown, NJ: Center for Family Life Education, 2005.

Taylor, Timothy. *The Prehistory of Sex.* New York: Bantam Books, 1996.

Williams, Linda. *Hardcore.* Berkeley, CA: University of California Press, 1989.

INDEX

About the Author

DR. MARTY KLEIN has been a Licensed Marriage and Family Therapist and Certified Sex Therapist for 31 years (that's over 30,000 sessions). His entire career has been aimed toward a single set of goals: telling the truth about sexuality, helping people feel sexually adequate and powerful, and supporting the healthy sexual expression and exploration of men and women.

Marty's six other books have been acclaimed by everyone from *USA Today* to *The California Therapist* to the Playboy Advisor, and are available in ten languages. A tireless speaker, Marty has given over 700 keynote speeches, training programs, and popular lectures across North America and 22 countries, including China, India, Croatia, Ukraine, Turkey, and Morocco. He estimates he has trained some 75,000 psychologists, physicians, social workers, nurses, and attorneys in human sexuality.

Marty has been honored by both the California Association of Marriage and Family Therapists and the Society for the Scientific Study of Sexuality. He has been an expert witness, consultant, or invited plaintiff in many state and federal trials involving censorship, obscenity, or other aspects of sexual expression. For 12 years he has written and published the electronic monthly *Sexual Intelligence* (www.SexualIntelligence.org), whose wit, passion, and research highlights the ways in which Americans' sexual rights are being challenged every day.

Marty's speaking schedule, original articles, extensive Q/A, and descriptions of his books and CDs are available on his Web site at www.SexEd.org. He can be reached at Klein@AmericasWarOnSex.com.

OTHER BOOKS BY MARTY KLEIN

Your Sexual Secrets:
When to Keep Them, When and How to Tell

Ask Me Anything:
Dr. Klein Answers the Sex Questions You'd *Love* to Ask

Let Me Count the Ways:
Discovering Great Sex Beyond Intercourse

Beyond Orgasm:
Dare to Be Honest About the Sex You Really Want

Sexual Intelligence:
What We Really Want from Sex, and How to Get It